CO-PUBLISHED WITH THE
AMERICAN ORGANIZATION OF
NURSE EXECUTIVES

Restructuring

THE IMPACT OF HOSPITAL ORGANIZATION ON NURSING LEADERSHIP

JOYCE C. CLIFFORD, PhD

press

American Hospital Publishing, Inc.
An American Hospital Association Company
CHICAGO

Cover design by Tim Kaage

Library of Congress Cataloging-in-Publication Data

Clifford, Joyce C.
  Restructuring : the impact of hospital organization on nursing leadership / by Joyce C. Clifford.
       p.   cm.
     "Copublished with the American Organization of Nurse Executives."
     Includes bibliographical references and index.
     ISBN 1-55648-229-9
     1. Nursing services—Administration—Case studies.   2. Integrated delivery of health care—Case studies.   3. Organizational change—Case studies.   I. American Organization of Nurse Executives.   II. Title.
     [DNLM: 1. Nursing Service, Hospital—organization & administration.   2. Hospital Restructuring.   3. Nurse Administrators.   4. Leadership. WY 105 C637r 1998]
RT89.C59 1998
362.1'73'068—dc21
DNLM/DLC
for Library of Congress   98-10015
                                                                                              CIP

Item Number: 177101

Contents

CHAPTER 7

Contextual and Thematic Findings

CHAPTER 8

Implications for the Future

About the Author

Joyce C. Clifford, PhD, RN, FAAN, is senior vice president for nursing and nurse-in-chief at Beth Israel Deaconess Medical Center in Boston and holds a visiting scholar appointment at Boston College School of Nursing. A graduate of St. Anselm College, she received her master's degree in nursing from the University of Alabama and her doctorate in the field of health planning and policy nursing at the Heller School of Brandeis University. She is a fellow of the American Academy of Nursing, a member and former president of the American Organization of Nurse Executives, and a member of the Robert Wood Johnson–sponsored Council on Economic Impact of Health Care Reform.

Ms. Clifford is an established author and consultant on the subject of organizational restructuring and the development of a professional practice model and has spoken both nationally and internationally on these subjects. In recognition of her contributions, she has received the American Hospital Association's Award of Honor in 1990, honorary doctorates from St. Anselm and Simmons Colleges and Indiana University, and numerous awards—including the national Sigma Theta Tau Dorothy Garrigus Founders Award for Promoting High Professional Standards, the Massachusetts Organization of Nurse Executives Award for Excellence in Nursing Administration, and in 1996 the American Organization of Nurse Executives' Leadership Award.

Forewords

T he entire health care system in the United States has undergone rapid changes in the last six years, and nowhere have the changes been more significant than in hospitals, particularly nonaffiliated independent institutions. Once considered the core of the health care system, these independent community and medical center facilities were strongly advised that if they wished to survive—let alone play a major role in the health care system of the future—they would have to completely restructure their operations or at the very least merge or consolidate with neighboring facilities to form larger hospital systems. Many institutions were advised to join large integrated health care systems, whereby the facility would be linked to prehospital and posthospital provider institutions. American hospitals took this advice to heart, and by 1996 the number of vertically integrated systems had grown to 566 and comprises almost 40 percent of all acute-care hospitals in the country.

The driving force behind these changes was a fundamental change in the way Americans pay for health care services. Where traditionally most health care services were paid by a private insurance company or the government on a fee-for-service basis, by the mid-1990s large capitated managed care plans were becoming the dominant form of coverage. These plans forced health care providers, especially hospitals, to reduce the prices they charged and to become part of systems that were capable of providing the full range of health care services to large employers whose employees required care to be available over a large geographic region. Efficiency and cost-effectiveness became the primary motivations for health care facilities in the '90s. On at least one measure, hospitals were successful in restructuring their operations. The cost of an average inpatient stay in an American hospital, which had been rising by 4 to 5 percent above inflation during the late 1980s and early 1990s, suddenly reversed course. Since 1994 the average cost of a hospital discharge has been growing 1 to 2 percent below inflation, actually registering a decline in real terms.

What these impressive findings fail to reveal, however, is that restructuring—if not accomplished with much care and understanding—can result in significant turmoil and confusion. These figures also hide the potentially negative impact such changes may be having on the quality of patient services available in the affected institutions. This book attempts to help remedy these shortcomings by taking us behind the scenes and vividly describing the impact of hospital restructuring on one of the most important components of the hospital workforce—its nursing staff.

Few individuals can match the credentials of Dr. Joyce Clifford, both in terms of bringing an in-depth knowledge of the day-to-day operations of a major nursing staff and having the perspective of an analyst trained in the broad area of health policy. The book's main focus is that nursing, and ultimately the quality of patient care, is strongly influenced by the existence of a chief nursing officer (CNO) and his or her leadership capabilities. Dr. Clifford's concern, which she documents in detail with three case studies, is that at times top management of a newly created hospital or integrated delivery system does not appreciate the unique role played by the CNO and may eliminate the position altogether. When this occurs, as it did in two of the case studies, nursing staff lose a sense of cohesiveness and direction, which might negatively affect patient care.

Restructuring: The Impact of Hospital Organization on Nursing Leadership also discusses the potentially detrimental effect of elevating a CNO to a more general adminstrative vice president position. While such a promotion might be viewed positively by the individual involved (although this is not always the case), the broader responsibilities that go with such a promotion redirect the focus of the individual away from the needs of the nursing staff. The nursing staff may feel that they have lost their leader and champion to the higher echelons of management.

The book also reveals another important lesson: that restructuring and the elimination of the CNO position are often associated with a deemphasis on clinical leadership; and if this occurs, it is likely to be detrimental to the quality of patient care. This is an important policy lesson that should be learned by all those involved in the restructuring of our health care system.

Lest readers think that the author is "stuck" in the past and against change, they will learn about the critical role that Dr. Clifford has assumed in the merging of two nationally recognized Harvard teaching hospitals. This book, therefore, is not simply an academic exercise, but rather a relevant study where the author gets to put into practice the lessons that she has learned through her scholarship.

—*Stuart H. Altman, PhD*
  Sol C. Chaikin Professor of National Health Policy
  at Heller Graduate School

T he notion of change is well established in health care, and the evidence of change fills a broad-banded spectrum. There is a litany of change that accompanies restructuring, reengineering, and regrouping, including major and minor structural changes and, most importantly, radical shifts in the roles and relationships of people in health care.

Restructuring: The Impact of Hospital Organization on Nursing Leadership is about how those changes have affected the role of the nurse executive. The reality of the situation is that no one group goes through any type of change alone. Although this book focuses on nursing, it is really about the changes in the way professional groups are organized in health care. Nurses are in a key pivotal role that collaborates and coordinates with both health care professionals and supporting staff. Any change in nursing, therefore, affects other health care disciplines, just as shifts in any other area affect nursing's ability to provide quality patient care.

Most past changes have been driven by efforts to improve quality. However, this improvement process can create "silos" of specialization, which keep people apart and can cause redundancy. The concept of continuous improvement means breaking out of these silos in order to create more integrated and interactive teams that share in goal setting and achieving results. In breaking down silos, departments have been dismantled and organizational work has been unbundled. The question presented in the book is, Are the resulting new structures achieving the mission better than the previous ones?

Historically, most of the health care professions built their standards of practice and care around the way the organization for health care delivery was structured—work processes were intertwined with the standards of care. Consideration of what any profession needs to do its work is important in change. The issue for the present is, To what extent have health care organizations diminished the capability of any professional group by unbundling or dismantling the structure? The issue for the future is to build on new knowledge and push for continuous improvement.

Dr. Clifford's book makes a major contribution to the field by bringing to life the experiences of selected groups in the midst of restructuring in health care delivery. The case studies along with the author's keen insights provide an understanding of how change is approached, as well as giving insight into the experience of restructuring and its effects on roles, relationships, and the ability to serve patients. The book provides a conceptual framework that can help organize change in nursing leadership. In addition, the author directs the reader beyond the present to consider the opportunities and the ramifications of how present actions affect the future of nursing.

Change is a way of life, especially in health care. This book has insights into restructuring and provides a platform for the next set of change iterations. In future change, the critical issue will be to form a new vision of what is critical to health professionals' roles and functions and what types of relationships best foster quality patient care—what type of organizational structure will position people for beneficial and productive relationships? These issues become increasingly complex because of the continual new discoveries and changes in patient-care technology. New technology allows for more "virtual" patient care while also accentuating the unremitting human need for care and compassion.

As you read *Restructuring: The Impact of Hospital Organization on Nursing Leadership,* consider that nurses have always contributed the heart to patient care; they have also contributed the wisdom of care planning and the continuity of care; and they have forged the standards and methods of quality patient care—and nursing has done all this in its characteristic unassuming and low-key way. These values need to be kept up and nurtured while facing the changes that the future most certainly will bring to health care.

　—Marjorie Beyers, Executive Director
　American Organization of Nurse Executives

Preface

Widespread restructuring and redesign of acute care delivery is taking place throughout the United States as hospitals attempt to reposition themselves in today's vastly different health care environment (Shortell, Gillies, and Devers 1995; Wunderlich, Sloan, and Davis 1996). Anticipating a future of severely reduced resources, hospitals now find it essential to undertake the formidable task of restructuring organizational relationships as a way to reduce costs and improve efficiency. In doing so, they are shifting away from the delivery of acute care services alone and becoming part of a larger, more integrated network of providers that share financial risk within a continuum of health services. Changing the hospital's focus from acute, inpatient services to community-based, ambulatory, and home health services has many implications for the future of both the organization itself and the delivery of patient care.

Bed reductions and employee downsizing are only two of the strategies being undertaken by hospitals to achieve their fiscal goals. Changing the skill mix of caregivers, reducing the number of hospital workers through cross-training, and developing interdisciplinary care teams with an integrated management system are other efforts under way to redesign the hospital's internal operations. Logically, these efforts are bringing about crucial changes in employment relationships within hospitals. Among the most potentially volatile internal operational changes are those that have begun to affect the traditionally strong employment relationship between hospitals and nurses.

For most of this century, hospital-based nursing services have been the primary practice setting for registered nurses and have served as the stage upon which professional nursing services have evolved and matured. Indeed, in large measure, development of nursing as a profession parallels development of the hospital as the major organizational structure in the U.S. health system. Acute care hospitals, in particular, have long been considered the hub of the health care system and inpatient, acute care settings have been viewed as the major practice settings for nurses. Moreover, the professional nurse, as described by Altman (1971, 1), has been considered the "backbone of the health industry." However, with the advent of managed care, integrated delivery systems (IDSs), and other major restructuring efforts aimed at reducing the use of expensive hospital services, hospitals are expected to lose their central role in the health care system as we approach the turn of the century. It stands to reason that a change of this magnitude will have a significant impact on all care providers, but probably no other group of health professionals will feel its impact more than nurses (Brannon 1994; *Hospitals* 1993). The current and expected shifts in the health care system have major implications for the planning and organization of nursing services.

As the current environment has brought about changes in the crucial relationship between hospitals and nurses, so too has it affected the relationships with, and the role of, the highest-ranking nurse, or senior nurse leader, referred to hereafter as the chief nursing officer (CNO). Because of the pivotal role nurses play in the delivery of health care, a study of the changing role of the CNO in the emerging hospital environment is essential.

PURPOSE OF THIS BOOK

This book describes a qualitative study whose primary purpose was to examine the CNO's evolving role in hospitals attempting to respond to a dramatically changed health care environment. The study was designed to explore how and why the CNO role is changing and to understand better the impact of that change on the management and administration of clinical nursing services. It was hoped that new paradigms for organizational change and managerial and professional leadership would emerge to support the development of IDSs and the changed environment for health care. The study involved multiple-site case studies, using interview, direct observation, and document review. Its results should prove useful to those charged with determining policy for health care organizations in the future.

A focus on the CNO's leadership responsibilities in the development of an organizational environment for the practice of nursing was chosen because of the growing body of literature that relates the design of nursing practice to the delivery of high-quality patient care (Aiken, Smith, and Lake 1994; Knaus et al. 1986; Shortell et al. 1994). Although patient care outcomes were beyond the scope of the study, the fact that the

CNO role is assumed to be an important organizational variable for patient care quality makes the study findings both important and policy relevant.

ORGANIZATION OF THE BOOK

This book consists of eight chapters and four appendixes. Chapter 1, "Nursing Services and Nursing Leadership in a Changing Hospital Environment," provides an overview and background of the role of nursing services in hospitals. Chapter 2, "A Review of the Literature," traces the professionalization of nursing and the evolution of hospital reliance on the nursing discipline. Chapter 3, "Study Approach," discusses the approach and research methodology used in this study. Three case studies are presented in chapters 4, "Red Hospital Case Study"; 5, "White Hospital Case Study"; and 6, "Blue Hospital Case Study." Chapter 7, "Contextual and Thematic Findings," describes the study's overall findings. And, finally, chapter 8, "Implications for the Future," summarizes the study and draws conclusions that may prove useful in preparing future hospital policy.

Acknowledgments

W here to begin seems to be a common question I encountered throughout the whole process of this research endeavor. Where to begin to study my area of interest; where to begin to analyze the rich data found; where to begin in developing meaningful conclusions—and now, where should I begin to acknowledge the tremendous support, guidance, direction, and general cheerleading I have received from so many during the process of developing my study interest and bringing it to this point of completion.

The first who comes to mind is my husband, Lawrence. Clearly, without his support and willingness to unselfishly give up the already limited personal time we have together, this dissertation would not have come to fruition. Larry's willingness to listen to endless renditions of the manuscript, and his suggestions for correction when I would start to get off track, were invaluable in keeping me focused. He is always an inspiration for me and I am so fortunate to have his continuing love, support, and encouragement.

Whenever I have been asked who was on my dissertation committee, my opening response is, "I have the best committee anyone could ask for." It's true. Led by committee chair Stuart Altman, PhD, the committee—consisting of Jon Chilingerian, PhD; Margaret McClure, EdD; and Constance Williams, PhD—could not have been a better combination. This was a team of experts and I am humbled by what I have learned from them. Stu Altman's unique perspectives from the policy and economic world were challenging for me, but led me always to a greater level of clarity. Jon Chilingerian's outstanding grasp of the organizational issues and his knowledge of the content of role and organizational theory provided me a framework for which I shall always be grateful. Connie Williams deserves a special thanks for helping me see the value of qualitative research as a way of developing my interests and for continuously motivating me through her keen insights and caring ways. Maggie McClure, a longtime friend and colleague, gave generously of her time, her special knowledge of the field, and her wonderful humor when I needed it the most. To each of them I will remain forever grateful.

I was given a special privilege by the CEOs and CNOs of the three hospitals I visited. They opened their doors for me, gave me access to their staff, and placed no obligations on me. At a time of great disruption in hospital organizations, they did not hesitate to share. I am extremely indebted to each of them for the trust they displayed. I hope that in their eyes, I have not misplaced that trust. I am also most grateful to the nursing management and other staff who participated in this study. They also took risks in sharing with me the complexities of the situations they are now encountering and their emotional strain as they try to respond professionally.

Without the support of my employer, the Beth Israel Deaconess Medical Center—and in particular Mitchell T. Rabkin, MD, and David Dolins—none of my doctoral work would have been undertaken. Their support, encouragement, and generosity of time are deeply appreciated.

I received an immense amount of support also from those with whom I work on a daily basis. The nursing management staff of the Beth Israel Deaconess Medical Center were magnificent cheerleaders for me— but most of all they inspired me to think about this topic, for they epitomize what can be achieved for patients, families, and communities when clinical leadership is effective. To each I express deep appreciation for giving me "distance" so I could complete this study.

There are other colleagues who should receive particular recognition for responding so often to my various requests, whether it was to help me edit, provide me a diagram that I did not know how to produce myself, advise me on methodology, or provide general assistance as I tried to balance a variety of competing activities. To each of the following I am extremely grateful: Laurie Leader; Deborah O'Connor; Margie Bachmann, RN; Kathy Horvath, RN; Jane Wandel, RN; Eileen Hodgman, RN; and Peter Buerhaus, PhD, RN, from the Harvard Nursing Research Institute.

Some colleagues served as readers for the unfolding story. Laura Avakian, senior vice president of human resources; and Peggy Reiley, RN, vice president of nursing at BI Deaconess; and two CNO colleagues, Yvonne Munn, MS, RN, and Trish Gibbons, DNSc, RN. Each provided invaluable insights. And, Marge Beyers, PhD, RN; Barbara Donaho, MA, RN; Beverly Henry, PhD, RN; along with Margaret McClure, EdD, RN, served as the expert panel who provided early assistance in helping me conceptualize the role changes of the CNO. I hope they find the results of this study useful.

I have been blessed with professional colleagues throughout the country and internationally, all of whom have provided me encouragement and I always promised I would say thanks to them as well. I am especially indebted to the work of Muriel Poulin, EdD, RN, whose career was devoted to the educational preparation for the CNO role. I hope this study indicates to her how much of a mentor she has served for me over the last two decades.

There is no way I can begin to express how important my assistant, Karen Poznick, was in bringing this paper to a close. She served as a gatekeeper of my time, scheduling opportunities for me to escape to the library or home to the computer; she became an expert in the format needed for the paper; she typed and proofread multiple versions of each chapter; and she gave up weekends and evenings to be sure that I would make deadlines. She was a true friend, encouraging me throughout. I am deeply appreciative for her unselfish extension of time and energy and thank her for really helping me to make this happen!

And, finally, I thank my close friend Jean Ahmann, who has really remained my motivation to get this paper done! To her, one of the best nurses I know, I dedicate this work.

1

Nursing Services and Nursing Leadership in a Changing Hospital Environment

I n the early twentieth century, the formation of diploma schools of nursing in hospitals provided hospitals with a steady supply of nursing labor. Many historians have viewed this development as a way for the hospitals of that era to ensure a constant, available source of cheap labor in the form of well-disciplined, young female workers who would accept subordinate autonomy to the hospital as well as to the usually male-dominated physician group (Reverby 1987; Rosenberg 1987; Seymer 1957; Starr 1982). By 1923 one-fourth of the 6,830 U.S. hospitals had their own school of nursing, and this number continued to grow through the 1960s (Reverby 1987).

At the same time, the professionalism of nursing was occurring, with nurses beginning to receive advanced education and greater recognition within the health field. Nurses began to use the hospital setting as a place in which to study and improve their practice and to advance their professionalism, thus creating a symbiotic relationship between nurses and hospitals and a strong employment alliance.

This chapter identifies the extent of the nursing workforce in today's hospitals and examines the effects on nursing services of hospital restructuring and redesign. It also looks at how the CNO role is changing and its impact on the delivery of patient care.

THE NURSING WORKFORCE WITHIN THE HOSPITAL

Although Rosenberg (1987) places the origin of modern nursing within the context of the mid-nineteenth-century hospital, the history of the trained nurse, now known as the registered nurse (RN), working in

1

large numbers within the hospital setting dates more precisely to the twentieth century and the Great Depression of 1929–1941 (Reverby 1987; Rosenberg 1987). Thus, for a large part of the twentieth century, hospitals have been the major employment setting for RNs in the United States. Throughout the past four decades, approximately two-thirds of the nation's RNs have been hospital employees. Even in the face of fluctuating supply and demand, the proportion of RNs working in hospitals has remained relatively constant. (See table 1-1.) And although the percentage of hospital-employed RNs declined somewhat after 1984, the actual number employed in hospitals continued to increase (Moses 1984, 1992).

The nursing department typically has represented about 40 percent of the hospital's total full-time equivalent employees (FTEs) and approximately 35 percent of the total hospital budget (Witt 1990). In sum, nursing services has customarily been the hospital's largest single department in terms of number of FTEs and budgeted salary and wages. The efficient management of these resources is vital for the hospital.

IMPACT OF RESTRUCTURING ON HOSPITAL NURSING SERVICES

As hospitals attempt to respond to an increasingly hostile financial environment, multiple efforts to restructure organizational relationships and approaches to the management of service delivery have been undertaken. Integrated networks of services are being developed, each attempting to reposition the role of the hospital within the network to become more cost-efficient and competitive in the anticipated financial environment of capitation and the growing managed care market (Shortell, Gillies, and Devers 1995). This response by hospitals holds

TABLE 1-1. Proportion of Hospital-Employed RNs to Number of RNs in the Workforce

	No. of RNs in Workforce	No. and Percentage of RNs in Hospitals
1962*	550,000	367,000 (66.8%)
1972*	780,000	578,000 (74.1%)
1984**	1,485,725	1,011,955 (68.1%)
1992**	1,853,024	1,232,717 (66.5%)
1996**	2,115,815	1,270,870 (00%)

*American Nurses Association, *Facts about Nursing, 1972–73.* Kansas City, MO: ANA, 1974. (Estimated numbers)
**National sample surveys of RNs (selected years)

far-reaching implications for the entire field of health care, but certainly clinicians, physicians, nurses, and other caregivers are feeling the immediate effect of these changes.

Because physicians have been recognized separately in the health care payment systems developed over the past 30 years, they, like hospitals, find themselves at the center of the national reform efforts and are recognized by all as major participants in the restructuring activities. Nurses, on the other hand, are hardly visible in any of the descriptions of new industry designs, even though they are the single largest group of health care professionals and an acknowledged critical element for the successful delivery of high-quality care (Koska 1989; Watson 1990, 1995). The phenomenon of nursing's invisibility in new industry designs is presumably due to at least the following four factors:

1. The strong identity of nurses as the main workforce of hospitals, with the implication that they are integrated into the overall discussions of hospital restructuring
2. The lack of independent financing that is specifically linked to nursing
3. The lack of a universal recognition of nursing as a discipline distinct from medicine
4. The perception that nursing, as a female profession, lacks professional autonomy in relation to the authority of the predominately male physician group

Ironically, although nursing as a professional discipline is noticeably absent from the discussion of network development, hospital restructuring efforts have had a strong impact on nurses and have begun to dramatically reshape the nature of nursing services in the hospital and elsewhere. Downsizing in hospitals has brought about reduced numbers of both bedside nursing staff and nurse managers. In Massachusetts alone, 19.7 percent fewer nursing administration and nursing management FTEs were reported for 1994 as compared to 1989 in a sample survey conducted by the Massachusetts Hospital Association (MHA) and the Massachusetts Organization of Nurse Executives (MONE) (MHA/MONE 1994). In a follow-up study of changes occurring between 1994 and 1995, in a matched sample of 50 acute care hospitals, the MHA reported a 5 percent decline in nursing administration positions and nearly a 14 percent decline in nursing management positions (MHA/MONE 1996). Although data related to bed closures in hospitals were not available at the time of this study, 48 of the 50 matched sample hospitals provided utilization data indicating a 5.1 percent decline in hospital discharges and a 9.8 percent decline in patient days. Some of the decline in nursing administration and nursing management positions may relate to the declining utilization of the hospital.

The power of the mass media has focused public attention on the issues of RN staff reductions in some hospitals and has raised questions related to the potential change in the quality of care provided (Colburn 1994; Kong 1994). Certain segments of the nursing community believe that the actions of hospitals, and therefore of hospital administrators and nurse executives, are detrimental to the practice of nursing and the care of patients (Cowley, Miller, and Hager 1995). In contrast, a 1996 report from the Institute of Medicine indicated that there is limited or no evidence to suggest that care outcomes have been affected by the restructuring and workforce reductions (Wunderlich, Sloan, and Davis 1996). What seems to be lost in this debate is any discussion of the potential impact of the changes occurring on the management and administration of nursing services and other clinical services as hospitals reposition themselves for a new era of limited resources.

THE CHANGING CNO ROLE

An examination of the CNO role in hospitals helps illuminate the importance of studying this role within the context of restructuring and redesign.[1] For the purpose of this study, a definition of the CNO was derived from the work of Poulin (1972) and Hunt (1994) as follows: "The CNO holds a senior administrative position in an organization. The CNO position is recognized as the official leadership role for nursing in the organization. Although incumbents may hold other administrative responsibilities, their primary role is the administration of, and leadership for, the nursing service. As a result of this set of responsibilities, the CNO is bound by a professional code of conduct as well as organizational expectations."

Perhaps more than most other senior positions in the hospital, the CNO position historically has been required to balance two sets of responsibilities: (1) as a senior member of the administrative and executive team, and (2) as the recognized professional leader of the major clinical discipline of nursing (Clifford 1981; Hunt 1994; Kelly 1977). As the senior manager, the CNO shares roles common to other managers. Ten such roles have been identified by Mintzberg (1973), who grouped them into three categories:

1. Interpersonal role (figurehead, liaison, leader)
2. Informational role (monitor, disseminator, spokesman)
3. Decisional role (entrepreneur, disturbance handler, resource allocator, and negotiator)

In the study described herein, these three groupings were used to categorize CNO organizational and professional responsibilities that were identified from the author's own CNO experience of nearly three decades and from a review of the literature. Not all ten roles were used in this matrix and, as Mintzberg points out, isolation of one role from another is somewhat unrealistic, for the work of the manager is integrated and separation by role activities is difficult to do. Nonetheless, a matrix of these roles in relation to CNO responsibilities was developed for the study and is shown in table 1-2.

Typically, it is the CNO who has responsibility for choreographing the direction of change for clinical nursing staff. This is the role considered essential in hospitals for the design of systems of nursing care delivery that are both qualitative and cost-effective and yet also provide professional satisfaction to nursing care providers. Integration of the goals of the professional discipline of nursing with the mission and goals of the health care organization is, in fact, the CNO's responsibility (Cilliers 1989; Clifford 1985). The intent of such integration is to maximize

- The quality of patient care
- The professional satisfaction of the nurse
- The goals of cost-effectiveness for the institution

It is the CNO who has had primary responsibility for ensuring an appropriately maintained balance among these three (Clifford 1981). Because nursing services are such a major part of the services provided in acute care settings, an interruption in the leadership required to achieve this balance could provide the organization with another level of risk.

Potential for Role Conflict

The potential for role conflict is noted especially in the CNO position. Traditionally, the CNO has been expected to function as a member of senior, and even executive, management to help the organization set and meet strategic goals. Often such goals are financially driven and frequently relate to the business strategies of the organization. When the CNO is an integral member of the executive team, a resource-driven approach to the development of care models for the delivery of nursing and other clinical services becomes better understood and accepted by the CNO. At the same time, as a member of the nursing profession, the CNO understands well the patient care needs approach traditionally used by physicians, nurses, and other clinicians as they plan and deliver care. Providing leadership in both of these organizational arenas is the balance the CNO must achieve when setting the direction for the design and management of nursing services within the organization. As a result, role conflict may be heightened for the CNO.

TABLE 1-2.   CNO Role Responsibilities: Organizational and Professional Components

Roles	Organization	Profession
• Interpersonal (Liaison, Integrator)	• Provides vision and direction for patient care • Provides leadership in the coordination of services • Integrates professional standards into system organization	• Provides clinical discipline leadership for continuing development of clinical excellence and care quality (research + evaluation) • Develops the environment for clinical practice by integrating professional and organizational goals • Mentors, sponsors, and develops nurse professionals
• Informational (Communicator)	• Brings a clinically based, patient-focused view to the business table of the organization • Interprets the mission, strategic direction, and business requirements to nurses and others, ensuring effective flow of information between executive and operational levels of the organization	• Interprets the nursing role in the health care system to multiple communities of the organization's internal and external environment • Establishes expectations for inter- and intradisciplinary collaboration
• Decisional (Designer)	• Is directly involved in planning and influencing the strategic direction mission and policies of the organization • Designs an organizational structure, systems, and standards for patient care delivery • Develops systems for evaluating the results of the care delivery system • Allocates and monitors resource utilization	• Defines nursing roles and evaluates system requirements for new roles (i.e., advanced practice) • Sets and meets professional standards for clinical care and nursing practice • Uses national standards of the profession in the redesign of the care delivery system

Moreover, members of the professional nursing staff hold high expectations that the CNO will provide leadership for the advancement of clinical practice and the development of the discipline of nursing (McClure 1989). This expectation may or may not call for more resources, but, more important, it relates to the way the CNO interacts and spends time with the nursing staff. As hospitals focus their attention on broader corporate goals, they expect their executive staff, including the CNO, to do the same. As the CNO becomes more business focused and spends more time on issues of the larger organization, the question arises as to whether there is the potential for an increase in what has been termed *professional-bureaucratic conflict* (Etzioni 1964). For those who have responsibility for providing leadership for a clinical discipline such as nursing, this potential raises important questions about the nature of their role in the changing hospital and health care environment.

Effects of Restructuring and Redesign on the Nursing Role

The prevalence of restructuring and redesign efforts in American hospitals is astounding, and the implications of the redesign trajectories hospitals are choosing are far-reaching in terms of effects on nursing practice and the organization of nursing services. In a 1995 survey sponsored by the Voluntary Hospital Association (VHA), Inc., 85 percent of all nurse leaders responding indicated that they have undertaken or are involved in a work restructuring or redesign project within their organization (VHA 1996). Many of these redesign efforts are based on the elements associated with patient-focused care (Lathrop 1991). Patient-focused care is one of the most popular models currently used for restructuring work in hospitals (Greiner 1995). Another of the models frequently used to gain efficiency in services and reduction in costs is operations improvement. In both models, the emphasis is on changing the skill mix of the nursing workforce, substituting less-skilled, usually unlicensed assisting personnel for the more costly RN. As hospitals develop the patient-focused approach to care delivery, there is a disaggregation of the typical departmental approach to professional and other patient care services. Patient services are blended in various ways through cross-training and the decentralization of many services to the patient care unit. The management structure needed to support this organizational design also differs from the traditional hierarchical and departmental approach typically found in hospitals. The integration of managerial roles is occurring, bringing substantive change to roles once considered impermeable.

In particular, major role change appears to be occurring in the position of the CNO in hospitals as work redesign and reorganization take place. Because these changes are currently in process, there is a dearth of literature describing the assorted patterns of role change. For the purposes of this study, a summary of the various patterns of role change thought to be occurring was developed. A panel of experts was used to confirm that these were the most dominant emerging patterns. (See chapter 3.) Table 1-3 summarizes the major patterns of change deemed to be currently under way.

These assumed patterns of change vary and range from elimination of the traditional CNO position in some organizations to a greatly expanded role in others, which might include areas beyond those related to the clinical discipline of nursing. In some circumstances, elimination of other nursing management positions occurs as well, resulting in a redesign of the conventional organizational reporting relationships of clinical nursing staff to administrators outside the discipline of nursing. In still other situations, cross-boundary responsibilities are being assumed by nurse managers and administrators at all levels of the organization.

Role Expansion

Role expansion is not new for the CNO. In the 1980s, it was associated primarily with the extension of responsibilities into the executive level of administration, bringing the CNO into full participation as a member of the senior level of management for strategic planning and program development for the organization (Kulbok 1982; Poulin 1984). It became an expectation that the CNO needed to be a member of the hospital's senior leadership team if the nursing department and the mission and goals of the larger organization were to be integrated (AHA 1983). Although this expansion of CNO role boundaries meant a larger administrative role in the organization, it did not necessarily mean that the CNO assumed operational accountability for the management of an array of other patient care services or for specific product lines, as became the case in the 1990s.

Now, as the CNO's administrative responsibilities are increased and the breadth of the role is expanded to cross department and other discipline boundaries, questions arise about the potential consequences of this change. Some believe that expanding the CNO role to include multiple other areas will increase the senior nurse executive's influence in positive ways; others suggest that expanding the boundaries beyond the areas associated with clinical nursing or the more direct care of patients dilutes the CNO role and prevents the development of strong leadership for nursing practice and thus for patient care; and still others suggest that the new design of health care services will not require a CNO and that the role will be eliminated or absorbed within another nursing position.[2]

There is some evidence to suggest that these changes in the configuration of nursing management are global in nature and not limited to the American hospital setting. Similar phenomena have been reported

TABLE 1-3. Patterns of CNO Role Change

Role	Pattern
• CNO changes career focus.	• Assumes an existing COO/CEO position; does not intend to remain as CNO or official professional nursing leader for the organization. A CNO position remains in the organization with someone else assuming the responsibilities.
• CNO role is expanded to include chief operating officer responsibilities.	• Incumbent continues as official professional leader for nursing; no other chief nursing officer role remains.
• CNO's administrative and senior professional leadership role continues.	• Performance expectations reflect responsiveness to changing environment (that is, concern for integrated system development and professional service design). CNO integrated into executive-level functioning of the organization.
• CNO moved to corporate level of the integrated or restructured delivery system.	• Some remain as the official professional nursing leader across the organization, assuming the overall professional leadership for care delivery management; others retain no continuing responsibility for care delivery management. Varied nursing leadership models in place at the discrete organizational levels of the system according to the nature of the corporate role.
• CNO role expanded to include line responsibilities for other patient care services and departments.	• Continues as the senior nursing leadership role in the organization; no other CNO role remains in organization.
• CNO role limited to internal management/administration of nursing department or to central professional support services for nursing staff.	• Is placed at department head level or senior administrative staff level organizationally, or position is eliminated as a separate position of the organization. Another nursing position assumes the designation of CNO and functions, when necessary, on behalf of the organization in this capacity (that is, to meet JCAHO standard)

in England, Scotland, Australia, and the Netherlands (Boyce 1992; Hunt 1994; Tribe and Campbell 1993). Moreover, in England, Australia, and New Zealand, the concept of general manager is being used more and more, and these managers are replacing professional managers in all disciplines, including nursing (Lowe 1994; News Analysis 1996).[3]

In addition, elimination of nursing administration positions or expansion of the functional responsibility of nurse administrators has a corollary in graduate nursing education. The Council on Graduate Education for Administration in Nursing (CGEAN) reports a reduction in nursing service administration graduate programs throughout the United States and has targeted this area as a strategic initiative for CGEAN nationally (Workman 1995).

It seems clear, then, that the restructuring of nursing administration and nursing management in hospitals arises from more than individual organizational decision making. Other, far-reaching phenomena are in place and need to be studied.

Two primary motivations for the redesign of the CNO position in hospitals are the overall reorganization taking place to move hospitals toward a network of health care services and factors directly related to cost-reduction strategies. Combining administrative role responsibilities or eliminating positions entirely may be viewed in some organizations as the appropriate way to achieve one or both of these reasons for change. However, whatever the underlying motivation for role redesign, the ultimate question is: What will this change, like so many others, mean for patient care? Are there consequences that relate to the quality of care provided? Because of the intrinsic nature of the CNO's relationship with clinical nursing staff, and consequently with patient care, redesigning or refocusing the CNO role raises important questions.

THE CNO'S IMPACT ON THE QUALITY OF PATIENT CARE

Strengthening the business focus of the senior leadership of the organization, including the clinical leadership in nursing and medicine, is not in and of itself the issue viewed as potentially problematic. Rather, it is the elimination or dilution of the nursing leadership role of the CNO position that may become troublesome. The important role of nursing leadership in designing systems of care delivery that both have good patient care outcomes and are professionally rewarding has been identified by many (McClure et al. 1983; Kramer and Schmalenberg 1988a, 1988b; Prescott 1993).

The author's personal experience suggests that the CNO role, when effectively carried out, helps the organization achieve its primary mission: high-quality patient care. Historically, the nature of nursing within the hospital is deeply embedded in the infrastructure of both care *and* management. Because of this, the work of nursing may simply be taken for granted, leading to a diminished understanding of the critical role nurses play in the hospital's overall effectiveness. It is the CNO's role to bring these contributions forward by designing, leading, and supporting effective systems of care delivery.

Indeed, the quality of organizational leadership, especially that related to nursing, has been identified as a significant organizational variable contributing to the caregivers' ability to achieve good patient care (Kramer and Schmalenberg 1988a, 1988b). Designing, implementing, and supporting systems that promote efficiency as well as quality are responsibilities of senior and executive nursing management. As discussed in more detail later, in the long run the quality of care provided by nurses can be related to the quality and effectiveness of nursing management (Aiken, Smith, and Lake 1994; Kramer and Schmalenberg 1988a). When hospitals undertake restructuring, failure to account for the impact of nursing management on outcomes associated with patient care, cost, and staff morale can only be viewed as a short-term focus in their efforts.

Systems of care delivery that failed to provide satisfaction for both patient and provider also have been identified as a major contributor to the two national nursing shortages reported in the early and late 1980s. The significant nature of the CNO's leadership role in the hospital organization was noted in the two national commissions that thoroughly examined the events contributing to these shortages (NCN 1983; DHHS 1988).

The report of the National Commission on Nursing (NCN) (1983) indicated what Aiken, Smith, and Lake (1994) later demonstrated in their research: The design of the nursing practice model provides nurses the opportunity to participate in clinical and other relevant organizational decision making that leads to improved nursing practice and high-quality patient care. And it is this design, or the crafting of an environment that supports professional nursing practice, that is the direct result of the leadership provided by the CNO. As indicated in the NCN report, "Nurses believe that the nurse administrators's participation in institutional policy development and planning directly influences their ability to provide quality patient care [p. 6]."

Further support for the notion that the environment for practice is crucial to patient care outcomes came from another report by Aiken on the relationship between the organization of nursing services and mortality rates in hospitals. In this study, Aiken found that the significant variables were not the number of RNs available for care but, rather, the level of nurse autonomy, nurses' control over their own practice, and nurses' relationships with physicians. These organizational factors were demonstrated in her study to be important variables related to decreased Medicare mortality rates in hospitals (Aiken, Smith, and Lake 1994).

These conditions for practice are directly related to the responsibilities the CNO has in designing an organizational and management system that supports and advances nursing practice. In the early 1980s, a serious national nursing shortage led the American Academy of Nursing to undertake a study of selected hospitals known for their recruitment and retention of nursing staff. These hospitals were referred to as *magnet hospitals*, a term still used to describe hospitals with attributes that support good nursing practice and high-quality patient care. Among the findings of *The Magnet Hospital Study* was the important role that nursing leadership has in designing and developing organizational models that support nurses in their ability to provide high-quality patient care (McClure et al. 1983).

Kramer and Hafner (1989) studied nurses in a subset of the magnet hospitals using an instrument known as the Nursing Work Index, in which respondents are asked to complete the statement "This is present in my current job situation" for a number of items related to the nurses' work environment and perceptions of patient care. Aiken, Smith, and Lake used the same instrument to derive the three scales they examined to measure the organizational outcomes of autonomy, greater nurse control over practice, and better relationships with physicians when selected magnet and nonmagnet hospitals were compared.

This author used the same instrument to prospectively identify items on the Nursing Work Index to develop a fourth scale called the Nursing Management Scale to measure the influence of nursing management on the environment in which nurses practice. Items used in the development of this scale included those that, for the most part, had not been used by Aiken in the development of the three scales used in her study.

An exploratory analysis, using factor analysis, confirmed that the items identified as representing nursing management are related and have properties that enable them to be used as one scale. The mean scores on the Nursing Management Scale were found to be significantly higher in magnet hospitals where nurses are known to have more autonomy, more control, and better relationships with physicians than in nonmagnet hospitals. No conclusions can be drawn from this preliminary study relating nursing management to lower mortality rates, nor has Aiken, as yet, demonstrated a causal link between autonomy, control, and relationships with physicians and mortality. However, the link between management and the intermediate organizational outcomes described by Aiken is strong in this exploratory analysis, supporting the theory that management works indirectly to influence patient outcomes by empowering nurses in their practice.

Thus, if management is an important variable in developing the conditions that lead to good nursing and possibly lower mortality rates, one of the critical elements that must be considered in the restructuring and redesign of new health care systems is what these changes do to the management and leadership of the nursing workforce. It becomes essential, then, to examine what is gained or lost as dramatic change takes place in the management system of nursing as viewed through the CNO role.

CONCLUSION

Hospital-based nursing services are at a critical juncture, facing major changes in their historical place within the hospital setting. The downsizing of hospital beds leads, subsequently, to a reduction in hospital staff. As the single largest department in the hospital, representing, on average, 43 percent of the hospital's labor force, nursing services are being placed in a vulnerable position by these events (Witt/Kieffer 1995). The hospital's nursing services cannot escape the budget reduction strategies of the organization or the restructuring and work redesign initiatives now being adopted throughout the United States. Included in these initiatives are the redesign and restructuring of nursing management and leadership roles. In many hospitals, the CNO role has undergone substantial change.

How the CNO role changes in response to the environmental factors influencing the hospital is important because of the central and critical role nursing has had in the organization. Important patient care outcomes are known to be related to the design of the nursing practice system, the responsibility for which resides mainly with the CNO. But also, the potential financial implications are high considering the level of budgetary responsibility assumed by the CNO. Ensuring cost-effective, high-quality patient care by designing, leading, and supporting professionally appropriate care delivery systems is the CNO's major role in the hospital. Changes in the expectations of this role have potential implications for the organization as a whole.

The CNO role has undergone considerable change over the past few decades. One major change is that CNOs are increasingly involved in the senior administration of the hospital while still managing and leading the professional department of nursing. Substantial change is taking place in this role, again with the patterns of change varying, it seems, according to organizational need. But one thing seems clear: Stability of the conventional CNO role is unlikely, and the changes that are already evident seem very divergent from each other. For some, change has meant elimination of the CNO role; for others, change has brought about an expansion of the CNO's responsibilities well beyond the discipline of nursing, crossing the boundaries of other disciplines and departments.

Notes

1. The term *chief nursing officer* (CNO) is used throughout this book rather than the other commonly used term of *chief nurse executive* (CNE). Although the descriptors for these roles often are interchangeable and have been considered the same in the recent past, the intent of the study was to learn more about the transformation of the senior nursing officer role, one aspect of which was to ascertain whether the role has achieved, maintained, or perhaps even lost executive role positioning and functioning during this time of turbulence in hospitals. Therefore, rather than presupposing executive-level practice by using CNE, the decision was made to use CNO unless it is clear that executive-level functioning was in place or intended.

2. This description of emerging patterns of the CNO role and the potential consequences of its change is based on many discussions with nurse executives throughout the country and CEOs in the field of hospital administration. It reflects opinions offered rather than evidence of outcomes.

3. Through personal correspondence and communication with colleagues in these countries, the author has learned that discipline-specific professionals as managers are being replaced by general managers without health care experience.

2

A Review of the Literature

A review of the pertinent literature encompasses many aspects of the organizational and professional dimensions of practice experienced by the CNO. Three major areas of review were undertaken for this study: (1) the organizational role that nursing and the CNO have had in hospitals traditionally and signs of its changing nature; (2) the changing health care system and specific factors affecting the hospital; and (3) organizational change theory incorporating the theoretical framework of role theory and the concept of professional-bureaucratic conflict and role ambiguity. This chapter examines these three areas of review.

NURSING AND THE TRADITIONAL ORGANIZATIONAL ROLE OF THE CNO

> Perhaps the most important single element in reshaping the day-to-day texture of hospital life was the professionalization of nursing. . . . Nursing, like professional hospital administration and changed modes of hospital financing, has played a key role in shaping the modern hospital (Rosenberg 1987, 8–9).

The important role that nursing has played in the development of the modern hospital is identified by others as well as Rosenberg. Starr (1982) likens the professionalization of nursing to the advent of aseptic surgery by Joseph Lister. These two developments, he indicates, can be considered responsible for the growth and character of the hospital industry in the United States. The development of three training schools for nurses in 1873, based on the Nightingale Schools in England, began the process that eventually led to hospitals' reliance on nurses to fulfill the increasingly complex responsibilities they were assuming.

Nightingale's Organization of Nursing Services

Florence Nightingale is well recognized as the founder of modern nursing as a result of the improvements she brought to the education and training of nurses in the latter part of the nineteenth century (Rosenberg 1987; Reverby 1987). However, her work on developing an administrative system for the organization of nursing services within the hospital, though spoken of less often, also is recognized as an important contribution in the development of hospital management systems (Henry, Woods, and Nagelkerk 1992; Palmer 1983).

Although numerous changes in the senior nursing officer role have occurred throughout the development of nursing in hospitals in the twentieth century, the die was cast for the way the CNO role would be developed when Nightingale presented her plan for the organization of the hospital (Woodham-Smith 1951). This plan has a remarkable resemblance to some of the tenets of organizational and management design now in place in many institutions throughout the United States. Of particular note is Nightingale's plan for a tripartite approach to senior management to include a lay administrator, a physician leader, and a senior nursing leader.

Nightingale also laid the foundation for the tradition of nurses managing nurses when she said that only those trained as nurses were qualified to govern or train other nurses (Woodham-Smith 1951). Seymer (1954) indicated that Nightingale assumed conflict would occur between the chief nurse and the lay administrator but that, in the end, the conflict would be a useful process in ensuring the improvement of patient care.

Nightingale's work established a legacy related to the CNO role that lasts until today. Dock and Stewart (1925) noted that it was her system that introduced the notion of superintendent of nurses to U.S. hospitals. They indicated that the head of the training school, which was attached to the hospital, had an important role in directing the educational program of the nursing students as well as managing the nursing department within the hospital. The early emphasis on the dual responsibilities of training and supervision for the senior nurse, who was called matron in the Nightingale system and superintendent of nurses in the American system (Seymer 1954), could be considered the forerunner of the two major dimensions typically considered inherent in the contemporary CNO role: advancing the practice of nursing and meeting the organizational requirements related to patient services (Cilliers 1989; Jeska 1994; Mauksch 1966; McClure 1989).

The Senior Nursing Role in the Twentieth Century

Throughout most of the first half of the twentieth century, the senior nursing officer role in U.S. hospitals resembled that discussed above.

There was a heavy emphasis on the training/educational responsibilities of the CNO with supervision of patient care being considered, in large part, as a dimension of the training of nurses, for it was student nurses who provided the major source of labor for hospitals (Starr 1982; Reverby 1987). It was Finer (1952), in a Kellogg Foundation research project carried out between 1950 and 1951, who examined the status of nursing administration in hospitals and, in particular, the role of the director of nursing.[1] Based on the study, Finer recommended that (1) nurses increase their knowledge of administration, (2) nursing services be coordinated with the top hospital management, and (3) further study be conducted on the relationship of hospital administrators and nursing directors.

In the decades since Finer's report, only sporadic interest has been shown in the examination of the CNO role in hospitals. A hiatus seems to have occurred in the 1960s and 1970s. In a review of nursing research between 1955 and 1968, Abdellah (1970) found no substantial studies related to the CNO role in hospitals. A review of *Dissertation Abstracts* indicates an increase in studies related to the CNO role beginning in the 1980s, perhaps because of the increasing emphasis on the CNO role in the changing hospital environment, and perhaps also because of the increase in the number of doctoral programs in nursing with a concentration on nursing administration. The leadership role of the CNO (Johnson 1981; Hyndman 1993; Tubbesing 1980), the education or competencies needed (Hansen 1993; McLemore and Hill 1965; Mullane 1959; Princeton 1993), the characteristics of CNOs (Cohen 1989; Jeska 1994), and the decision making of effective nurse leaders (Lumley 1988; Wangsness 1991) appear to be the most common topics studied in relation to the CNO position in hospitals.

In a study of the relationship of the organizational culture and the leadership effectiveness of the nurse executive, Davis (1989) found that the greatest cultural influence on the CNO was the profession of nursing itself and not the organizational setting. This is an important finding that Davis suggested might indicate that the CNOs studied were effective nurse leaders but not necessarily effective organizational leaders. Wangsness (1991) found that nurse executives were very much involved in organizational-level decision making, especially as it related to quality assurance activities. An additional finding in the Wangsness study was that the CNO had much autonomy in the decisions that related to the department of nursing. It could be extrapolated from this study that the professional dimension of the CNO role was present as was the organizational dimension.

Organizational-level placement of the director of nursing (CNO) in 20 Air Force hospitals was studied by Burner (1983) to determine whether this placement made a difference in the CNO's ability to promote safe, competent care for patients. The study conclusions indicated that organizational placement of the CNO had an effect in two areas: the nurse-physician relationships, and the safety and competence of nursing care.

Poulin's Studies of the CNO Role

It is the work of Poulin (1972, 1984) that provides the greatest insight into the structure and function of the CNO role. In a 1972 dissertation study, she examined the nursing service administrator role (CNO) for purposes of ultimately planning graduate programs for its preparation. Poulin's findings led her to conclude that the CNO's scope of responsibility was moving away from an internal focus, leading the CNO into a complex pattern of interactions. Placement of the CNO in the organizational hierarchy influenced this pattern as well. Poulin predicted that the CNO role would become more of a coordinating role within the department of nursing as nursing increased its professionalism. And, finally, Poulin's study suggested that the context for potential conflict was present as the administrative demands of the organization increased and were juxtaposed with an increasing focus within the nursing profession on clinical practice.

In 1980 Poulin replicated this study. Changes similar to those predicted in the 1972 study were found, especially as they related to the scope and responsibility of the nurse administrator and placement in the organization. Increasing responsibilities across patient care departments and into the broader community were evident. The nurse administrator of 1980 also was more apt to be at the senior level of management in the organization (Poulin 1984). Poulin indicated that an important question needing study was: What will be relinquished as the role changes, and what are the implications for the organization as the job expands for the CNO? It appears that no other research study has attempted to look at the implications of the CNO's expanding role in the hospital. In part, the study described in this book begins to answer the question Poulin raised in her 1984 study.

CNO Inclusion in the Hospital's Executive Leadership

The senior leadership position for nursing in hospitals has not always held executive-level positioning. The continuing development of the director of nurses (as the CNO was most likely to be called) as an active member of hospital management took on new meaning following development of prospective payment systems (PPSs) for hospitals with the use of diagnosis-related groups (DRGs) in the early part of the 1980s. An increased emphasis on the business management of the institution gave new direction to the CNO. Prior to this time, many CNOs often were not even involved in the development of the budget for their own department, let alone involved in the strategic planning for the hospital as a whole (ASNSA 1977).

The work of the American Society for Nursing Service Administrators (ASNSA), an organization established in 1967 as an affiliate of the American Hospital Association (AHA), was instrumental in helping develop the role of the director of nursing as a member of the senior administrative team in the hospital. It was the efforts of the leadership of this organization, now known as the American Organization of Nurse Executives (AONE), in the late 1970s and early 1980s that convinced members of AHA's leadership of the importance of having the CNO at the executive level of the organization. J. Alexander McMahon, then president of the AHA, was very influential in establishing the standard calling for the CNO to be a member of the executive leadership team in hospitals.[2] This standard became more specifically recognized in the AHA document *Future Directions* (1983), which was developed by the board of trustees to provide strategic direction to the organization: "The members of the executive management team [in hospitals] are those designated by the CEO. The selection of members will vary depending on the particular circumstances of the hospital. In its discussions, however, the Board considered nursing administration as part of executive management [p. 9]."

The initiatives of the AHA and its affiliate, the ASNSA, paralleled other work taking place in the early to mid-1980s. Serious nursing shortages during this period led to establishment of a National Commission on Nursing (NCN) sponsored by the AHA and the American Hospital Supply Co. The commission's *Summary Report and Recommendations* (1983) received much visibility because of the commission's multidisciplinary nature and the high credibility within the hospital field of many of its members. Their recommendation, in 1983, for nursing to be involved in policy development and decision making throughout the organization was especially important in motivating change in the design of nursing services throughout the hospital industry and in bringing the CNO position to the executive management team in many hospitals.

THE CHANGING HEALTH CARE SYSTEM

The literature clearly shows that the environment for health care is quite different today than ever before. Competition among health care institutions is increasing, work redesign and hospital restructuring is expected, and, as Ryan (1990) indicated, the health care system is moving from procedure-bound organizations to organizations that promote, measure, and reward quality outcomes and effectiveness. This corresponds with the work of Kanter (1989), who noted the need for managers to create environments that hold high-quality care, people, and the bottom line on equal status. Sovie (1995) offered an inventory of restructuring ideas from university teaching hospitals indicating that only time will tell which of these will yield the desired outcomes—those that will create the environment outlined by Kanter.

Changes in Hospital Financing and Structure

Changes in hospital financing (DRGs, managed care, and increasing capitation, specifically) have had an impact on the CNO's work and the design of management and care delivery systems in the hospital. The move to a PPS resulting from the Tax Equity and Fiscal Responsibility Act of 1982 (TEFRA) began a change that continues today in the way that hospitals approach the business of providing services. Davis, Powell, and Gross (1987) noted that the incentive of the PPS to decrease length of stay (LOS) increases the likelihood that patients will require more home care and skilled nursing services following discharge from the acute care hospital. Studies by Carroll and Erwin (1987) were unable to demonstrate an increase in utilization of long-term care facilities following implementation of a PPS, but a change in the level of care requirements of those admitted to the long-term care facility was experienced.

In a discussion of the implications of PPSs for nursing, Jones (1989) suggested that the evolution of this payment system into a fully capitated, managed care system might bring with it greater support for the use of the advanced practice nurse (APN). Some consider this staffing strategy as a potential way to offset the decrease in the number of staff available to patients by providing more expert practitioners to assess and plan patient care in an efficient manner. Jones also discussed the important role the CNO has in developing methods for evaluating the financial impact of staffing decisions such as this.

Of five trends identified in a 1992 State Health Reform report (*Hospitals* 1992), managed care was considered the leading cost-containment initiative influencing hospitals. Managed care, as defined by the Society for Ambulatory Care Professionals (1994), relates to the control of access, cost, and/or quality of the health care provided. This is accomplished by the management of diagnosis, treatment, or the use of procedures either prior to or at the time of the delivery of services. Managed care organizations (MCOs), the most common of which is the health maintenance organization (HMO), rely on discounted fees or capitation to achieve the goal of reducing the amount of health services provided (Buerhaus 1996). The move toward increased managed care places heavy emphasis on primary care services, health promotion, and health maintenance through primary care physician practices and neighborhood or other health center settings in the community. A reduction in both the size of the hospital and the services provided is the result of this change to community-focused care delivery (Shortell, Gillies, Anderson et al. 1993).

The development of integrated delivery systems (IDSs) suggests that there will be a redistribution of services in the future. The conventional hospital-based or inpatient-focused acute care services, long considered the core of the health care system in the United States, are expected, in large part, to be replaced with community, ambulatory, and home care services (Shortell, Gillies, and Devers 1995). The goal of an IDS is to achieve economic and clinical integration vertically in an effort to improve the coordination of services while reducing costs. Development of these systems usually includes the affiliation of hospitals, physicians, and other community health agencies that form a network for coordinating and delivering a broad range of services to the community considered the market for the IDS (AHA 1994).

Changes in Hospital Work Activity

Numerous other authors discuss the multitude of changes now being experienced by hospitals. Decreases in LOS, reduction in the number of beds, development of case management systems, and product line/service line management are but a few changes discussed. *Product line restructuring* refers to the trend in hospitals today to use the concept popular in business to develop strategic business units around similar groups of clinical services. In this model, the management structure is decentralized and total authority is given to the manager for the entire product line, sometimes referred to as a *clinical service line*.

As previously noted, patient-focused care is among the most popular of the changes considered by some as a way for hospitals to refocus their inpatient work activity (Greiner 1995; Lathrop 1991). In this care delivery model, the locations of services, including diagnostic services, are placed as close as possible to the patient. This decentralization of services to the site of care delivery, whenever possible, leads to other changes as well. Cross-training is used to develop multiskilled workers and places management of these workers as well as multiple clinical disciplines under the leadership of one manager, often the nurse manager. This usually means a reduction in the use of RNs, although there is an expectation for increased interdisciplinary planning for patient care. Central to the theme of patient-focused care is the notion that continuity of care, coordination, and integration will occur among health professionals and caregivers, eliminating boundaries or barriers to the person receiving the care.

This thought, postulated by Gilmore, Hirschorn, and O'Connor (1994) as well as others (Ashekenas et al. 1995), forms the basis for the consideration of new organizational designs in the developing integrated health care system. Gilmore, Hirschorn, and O'Connor proposed four new boundaries for organizations related to authority, tasks, politics, and identity. They suggested that health care leaders must develop boundary competence in order to function in a more open, flexible, and multidisciplined setting (71). The points raised in this discussion have relevance for the CNO redesigning the work elements for collaborative relationships in the future.

Bergman (1993) considered the health care system of the twenty-first century, envisioning that the hospital will be viewed no longer as a "place" but, rather, as a "system" with different programs dispersed over a large geographic area, which would eliminate the traditional approach of bringing all acute care systems under a single roof called the hospital. This vision of the future hospital with health care services dispersed raises important questions about the way such services will be organized and the way the health care workforce will be designed.

Robinson (1994) spoke of boundaries in relation to the hospital, indicating that fundamental change is occurring in these traditional organizations. The expansion of hospital services into ambulatory, subacute, home care, and other, more diversified activities is expected to accelerate, and more vertically integrated systems are expected to emerge.

Berwick (1994) argued that there is more rhetoric to the discussions of health care reform than actual change. He suggested that the change experienced is in regulations, payment, and corporate structures, not in those things that will improve the health status of individuals. Berwick challenged clinicians, physicians, nurses, and others to accept more responsibility for change, adding that by doing so they will feel more in control than is currently the case.

ASNSA/AONE Surveys Showing the Impact of These Changes on the CNO Role

A series of surveys by ASNSA/AONE illustrate how some of these changes have affected the CNO role. Beginning in 1977, ASNSA members began to participate in what has become a periodic survey of their role, scope of responsibility, and practice environment. Two surveys (1977 and 1982) were carried out solely by ASNSA. In 1986 Witt Associates, a management recruiting firm, took on the responsibility of surveying AONE members. The subsequent three surveys, in 1988, 1990, and 1994, were cosponsored by AONE. A review of the survey results provides an interesting profile of how some aspects of the CNO role have continued to change. Table 2-1 demonstrates the change in position title, an indication of organizational placement of the CNO over this period of time.

The most significant change noted is a decline in the use of the title director of nursing, a title that is presumed to connote department head rather than executive-level placement in the organization. Although in each year of the survey the questions were posed somewhat differently, the decline in use of this title and the upswing in use of the corporate title of vice president following implementation of PPSs in hospitals are not likely due to the survey tool. The 1994 survey results, although indicating that use of the vice president title was increasing, also showed that use of the title vice president for patient care services was growing in popularity (Witt/Kieffer 1995). This change in title coincides with the finding in this same survey that 81 percent of those responding indicated they have had a change in responsibilities over the past two years. A review of the areas identified by the respondents suggests (1) an expansion of responsibilities to incorporate long-term care and home care services, and (2) an increase in responsibilities related to other professional and clinical services as well as support and hotel services. Table 2-2 displays changes occurring in resources managed by the CNO. Of interest is the increase in FTEs under CNO responsibility in 1994, again representing the change to an integrated patient care service under CNO management.

In the 1986, 1988, and 1990 surveys, the FTEs reported and shown in table 2-2 are identified in the reports as nursing FTEs. For 1994 the FTEs and budgets reported are identified as representing patient care

TABLE 2-1. Organizational Titles Reported by CNOs

Titles Reported	1977	1982	1986	1988	1990	1994
Associate administrator/ senior vice president	1.3%		9%	13%		16%
Vice president of nursing/ patient services	1.6%	17%	49%	62%	61%	68%
Assistant administrator		19%	15%	11%	11%	
Director of nursing	77%	37%	26%	14%	11%	11%
Other		10%				23%

TABLE 2-2. CNO Responsibility: Ratio of Budget and FTEs to Overall Hospital

	1986	1988	1990	1994*
FTEs as percentage of hospital total:	41%	38%	40%	43%
Budget as percentage of hospital total:	32%	33%	35%	33%

*Includes those hospitals reporting an integrated patient care service.

services. No attempt to report nursing FTEs alone was made in the 1994 report. However, the 1994 report highlighted that "the typical patient care department has a dominance of RNs [and] uses cross-trained workers." (Witt/Kieffer 1995, 10). The increase in use of lower-paid, unlicensed personnel and the cross-training of both licensed and unlicensed staff may account for the stability of the ratio of budget-to-hospital total when, at the same time, the ratio of FTEs-to-hospital total has increased. Caution must be exercised in drawing conclusions from these surveys, which report averages of the responses returned.

Although the studies conducted from 1986 on by Witt and Associates did not report the extent of CNO involvement in budgetary activities for the hospital and the nursing department, the first two surveys by ASNSA showed the lack of involvement of this senior member of the management team in hospital and even department budget planning prior to PPS implementation. Table 2-3 shows these findings on the CNO responsibility in the planning and administration of budgets.

Again, these data suggest the increasing accountability the CNO has assumed over the past two decades. The 1977 data show that a relatively low percentage of the CNO respondents were fully involved in the budgetary process for either the hospital or their own area of responsibility, the department of nursing (ASNSA 1977; ASNSA 1982). Clearly, the level of participation changed at both levels of the organization—the hospital as a whole and the department—by the time of the 1982 survey. Also, the change between surveys in the CNO's administrative responsibility for managing the nursing budget suggests that the increased involvement of the CNO in hospital and departmentwide financial management was accompanied by an increase in autonomy and accountability within each CNO's area of responsibility. It is assumed that budget involvement now is such a basic component of CNO responsibilities that it no longer is considered a significant question for the survey.

Other findings in these surveys suggesting that change is occurring in the hospital organization and CNO responsibilities include the beginning signs in 1990 of managerial downsizing, with 59 percent of CNOs reporting they had eliminated director or supervisory positions (Witt Associates 1990). CNO reporting relationships also changed in 1994, with 60 percent reporting to the CEO, an increase over previous surveys that reportedly is due to elimination of the chief operating officer (COO)

TABLE 2-3. CNO Involvement in Budget Process

	1977	1982
Participates in hospital budget	51%	83%
Participates in nursing budget	73%	93%
Administrative responsibility for nursing budget	56%	86%

position in some hospitals or incorporation of these responsibilities into the CNO position.

Further signs of change for both the hospital organization and the CNO were reported for the first time in the 1994 survey. Thirty-seven percent of the respondents reported they had experienced a merger or affiliation in the past two years, so-called corporate duties were reported by 14 percent of the CNOs, and managed care as a percentage of total revenues was reported for the first time. Finally, the 1994 survey reported, for the first time, that severance agreements were part of the CNO work agreements. Although the data indicate that only 24 percent of the respondents have such an agreement, Witt Associates reported that this finding may relate to the seniority of the incumbents because "all of the CNOs they have placed in recent times have a severance agreement" (Witt/Kieffer 1995). This change to negotiated severance contracts at the time of employment suggests that the CNO position is recognized as part of the senior management level of the organization whose employment is considered to be at high risk in the current environment of hospital mergers, downsizing, and more stringent financial goals.

As viewed through the survey reports of Witt Associates and the AONE, change in the CNO role has been occurring over the past decade and a half. As CNOs became more involved in senior-level management in hospitals, their responsibilities for finance and strategic planning were enhanced. The need for the nurse executive to assume these responsibilities while also exercising leadership for the professional dimensions of the role is supported by John Colloton, who, in 1984, as director of the University of Iowa Hospitals and Clinics, advanced four challenges to the nurse executive of the future. Speaking to the Boston University graduates of the Commonwealth Fund Executive Nurse Leadership Program, Colloton indicated that

- Nurse executives must understand and prepare to influence and cope with the dramatically changing environment in which their health care organization must operate.
- The nurse executive is challenged to develop and sustain a practice environment for nurses that nourishes high staff morale and high-quality patient care in a climate of revolutionary change and shrinking resources.
- The nurse executive must maintain and strengthen professional relationships within the changing health system to the end of rendering the highest quality patient care within available resources.
- The nurse executive must become fully committed to and engaged in strategic planning on an institutionwide level.

Although Colloton's discussion was motivated in large part by the changes in hospitals brought on by the advent of PPSs in the first half of the 1980s, their relevance to present-day nurse executive practice was confirmed by the expert panel used in the study described in this book. (See chapter 3.)

Response of Organized Nursing to Hospital Restructuring

Workplace restructuring and job redesign efforts impact the health care organization in many ways. For example, these changes have spurred union-organizing activities in a number of institutions. Issues related to union organization have been of concern to hospitals for many reasons. Chief among these is the potential interruption of patient care activities because efforts become directed toward contract negotiation and other union-related activities. Moreover, continuous bargaining with an outside agent not committed to the organization's goals and mission is not considered an efficient use of important hospital resources. In general, all attempts are made to avoid having employees, especially nursing staff, unionize. A 1995 report of the American Society of Healthcare Human Resource Administrators (ASHHRA) indicated that an upswing in union activity was reported from one six-month period (July–December 1994) to the next (January–June 1995), with RNs among those targeted for union activity. At 29.6 percent (in 56 hospitals), RNs represented the largest single group targeted. The issues of job security, staffing, and quality of care were identified as the first, second, and fourth concerns given as reasons for the increased interest in unionization. Workplace restructuring and job redesign were cited as having an impact on this issue.

Job redesign for nursing has two dimensions: the most efficient use of professional staff and a change in skill mix. In the first case, there is the need to ensure that the more expensive professional staff are not used to perform functions that can be easily performed by less-skilled personnel, such as transporting patients to areas off the clinical unit or distributing food trays and supplies to patient rooms. In an article on the future of hospital nursing, Aiken (1990a) commented on the dissatisfaction nurses have when they must perform nonnursing functions that could be accomplished by members of a hospital's nonclinical support services. Again, on the subject of restructuring, Aiken (1990b, 23), in a letter to the editor of *Health Management Quarterly*, wrote: "We have no substitute for human caring. Our agenda for the '90s must include creative strategies to restructure health-care settings to make them more attractive places to work. Competitive compensation is needed, but the power of intrinsic rewards should not be underestimated."

For most nurses, "intrinsic rewards" include the ability to provide high-quality patient care and the opportunity to work with competent colleagues (Kramer and Schmalenberg 1988b). These are two areas now viewed by many nurses as being at risk as downsizing and changes in the skill mix of hospital workers take place (Cowley, Miller, and Hager 1995).

The change in skill mix referred to in this context is the second dimension of job redesign in nursing. Many nurses are expressing concern about the reported increased use of nonlicensed staff to perform clinical functions for patients generally considered by nurses to be their responsibility. In an atmosphere of downsizing in hospitals, the de-skilling of the workforce is considered a critically important issue, one that ultimately relates to the quality of patient care (Twedt 1996).

The Changing Nature of the Business of the Hospital

Hospitals, and health care organizations in general, have been considered "professional organizations," or organizations that rely heavily on specialists or professionals to establish the standards around which the coordination of needed activities occurs. The division of labor into tasks to be accomplished and the coordination of those tasks defines the structure of an organization, according to organizational theorist Mintzberg (1989). Professionals usually are recognized for having a unique body of knowledge acquired through formal training undertaken in their area of specialization. Their standardized knowledge and skill are coupled with individual discretionary judgment, allowing them to maintain control over their own work.

The hospital has been influenced for most of this century by two dominant professions, medicine and nursing. However, as restructuring and redesign proceed, will hospitals remain "professional" organizations as defined by Mintzberg, or will they behave and respond more and more like business corporations? And if the latter is true, does this raise questions about the kind and quality of leadership needed for a restructured health care environment? For the purposes of the study described in this book, this question is raised specifically as it relates to the administration and management of the nursing services in an environment of change.

Learning more about the way organizations change is an important component of the study. Hurst (1995) put forth a model of organizational transition that speaks to the differences between young and mature organizations. Young organizations are apt to be in the learning cycle of change; mature organizations move into a cycle of performance. Although these concepts, learning and performance, may be at two ends of the continuum, Hurst noted that all organizations include some of each. Hurst also addressed the need for organizations to adopt a "values-based rationality for change" (7), arguing that action taken intentionally as part of the process of change should be carried out because it is intrinsically valuable. Maintaining a focus on mission and a central set of values establishes a means for all members of the organization to take action and move forward (39). This approach to organizational change has relevance for the hospital because of the large number of professionals who hold many similar values on quality of care and professional autonomy.

The concept of a profession-oriented organization also was discussed by Benveniste (1987). Benveniste identified three distinct characteristics of the professional organization (257):

1. A large number of professionals are employed and engaged in the core activities of the organization.
2. Managers and professionals have a higher level of interdependence, sharing information in a more direct way.
3. Controls within the organization are more likely to come from professional discretion and self-regulation.

Change in the profession-oriented organization is more likely to come from intrinsic motivators and emphasis on conflict resolution.

Physicians and the Management of Organizations

Changes in economic incentives for physicians, coupled with their concern for clinical service outcomes, have led to the increasing involvement of physicians in the governance and administration or management of health care organizations, including hospitals. This is evidenced in part by the growing membership in the American College of Physician Executives, which increased by 3,000 members over a five-year period (Sherer 1993). A similar trend has been noted by the American Academy of Medical Directors (Sherer 1993). To a large extent, the increased involvement of physicians in organizational management is in response to the intrusion they perceive as others scrutinize their clinical judgments (Davidson, McCollum, and Heieke 1996).

Recognizing the different types of decisions physicians and managers control, Dunham, Kinkig, and Schulz (1994) researched the perceived value of physician executives in the organization. They found that both physicians and nonphysician hospital administrators believe that the involvement of physicians in organizational decision making was of value. Tjosvold and MacPherson (1996) studied the interdependence of the physician and nurse administrator roles as it relates to the theory of competition and cooperation. They found that the way these two clinically based administrators interacted was of importance in the organization's effectiveness and the hospital's capacity to improve care. Both these studies have significance for the changing role of the CNO in hospitals and the future role relationships the CNO will have with physician executives and managers.

ROLE RELATIONSHIPS WITHIN ORGANIZATIONS

To study how organizations function, it is important to understand the concepts of role and status. *Role* generally is defined as an organized set of behaviors identified with a position. It encompasses both the expectations of behavior for a specific role as well as the behaviors actually being performed by the incumbent in that role (Christman and Counte 1981; Mintzberg 1989; Newcomb, Turner, and Converse 1965). The notion of organizational *status* expands the concept of role by suggesting a hierarchical relationship among roles, with some being more prestigious than others. This leads to the development of social structures and social stratification within the organization. Individuals often cross over multiple social structures within the organization and must adjust their role behaviors to meet the expectations of each structure (Georgopoulos 1972).

The Influence of Structure on Role

Mumford and Skipper (1967) suggested that structure influences how individuals are able to carry out their roles in an organization. They indicated that organizational positions appear in clusters. Some sociologists have described these clusters as role sets or role partners (Merton 1957; Newcomb, Turner, and Converse 1965). Role partners interact with each other and hold expectations for the person in the role based on position, title, and other evidence of who they are or what their status is in the organization. Sets of role partners occur and privileges are granted to one set that may not be granted to another. This is especially so with regard to information exchange, the sharing of ideas, or helping one another solve problems. The way one is perceived in the role shapes the role partners and the relationships that occur (Christman and Counte 1981; Merton 1968).

The notion of role partners is especially relevant to the CNO in hospital organizations who, perhaps even more than others in senior management positions, is expected to coordinate and integrate services across departmental lines, or across role partner sets. To accomplish this integrating function, the CNO position must be structured so that both formal and informal means can be used to interact and share expectations with role partners (Newcomb, Turner, and Converse 1965). That is, there must be similar role status. In a seminal study of the work of managers, Mintzberg (1973) identified and categorized a set of ten roles representing common activities of all managers. (See chapter 1.) Regardless of where they are placed in an organization, managers are responsible for managing the boundaries between their areas of responsibility and the larger environment. A common set of managerial roles is used by managers to accomplish this, leading Mintzberg to argue that there are common characteristics to the work of all managers.

Professional-Bureaucratic Conflict and Role Ambiguity

Given the complexity of most organizations and the opportunity for any one individual to have multiple role sets, Blau and Scott (1962) suggested that it is not surprising that role conflict occurs. Newcomb, Turner, and Converse describe role conflict as follows (417): "Role conflict arises not just because of doing different or opposite things in assuming different role relationships. . . . The crux of the matter lies, rather, in the fact that any role relationship involves at least two persons, each of whom has a set of expectations concerning each of them. Role conflict stems from these expectations—either because role partners have contradictory ones or because those of one partner are unwelcome to the other." When it occurs in clinical or professional roles within the hospital organization, role conflict often extends to the phenomenon commonly referred to as professional-bureaucratic conflict.

Through a managed competition approach, the payer has gained significant ground in directing and shaping, from its business-oriented perspective, the provision of health care services. Clinicians, especially physicians and nurses, often indicate they feel out of the loop in these decisions. Worse, they fear a loss of professional autonomy, traditionally a major hallmark of the professional role. They express concern about the impact of payers' decisions and subsequent organizational changes on (1) the outcomes of patient care and (2) their ability to exert their authority as professionals in rendering decisions that relate to clinical care and programs of service.

Etzioni (1969) described professional-bureaucratic conflict as a major concern for the professional organization, suggesting that "the authority of knowledge and the authority of administrative hierarchy are basically incompatible" (viii). Throughout the past two decades, various forms of organizational management have been implemented in an attempt to decrease this conflict potential. Crossley (1993) found that the involvement of nurses at the executive level of the organization was helpful. The current integration of physicians into the management structure of hospitals, through either formal means or various committee and information-sharing processes, is another attempt to diffuse the potential for conflict. Also, the development of physician-hospital organizations (PHOs) is intended to integrate physicians into the management structure of the hospital, in part to help diffuse the potential for conflict in the current environment. Similar organizational models do not exist for nursing and its relationship with the hospital because nursing has always been a part of hospital administration. However, as nurses have developed a stronger professional identity and a sense of autonomy as members of a clinical department, the potential for role conflict within an environment of hospital downsizing becomes increasingly important. Thus, as hospitals change their organizational structures, as they respond to the financial directives of payers, and as they behave more like corporations seeking to increase their revenue margins, the question of professional-bureaucratic conflict and its consequences on the future design of health care systems becomes increasingly relevant.

In a study by Tucker (1992), issues related to moral reasoning and the decision making of chief nurse executives was explored. Among the findings was that nurse executives face many dilemmas in their work, but the most frequently encountered ethical dilemma concerns resource allocation and quality of care. Tucker viewed this as part of the traditional, goal-driven professional ethos up against a resource-driven model of decision making. Crossley (1993) studied the level of role conflict and role ambiguity in the CNO role and the access or proximity the CNO had with the governing body of the organization. Based on the theory that direct access reduces role conflict and clarifies ambiguity, Crossley's findings demonstrated a consistent decline in role ambiguity for those CNOs who were in close proximity to the organization's governing body.

CONCLUSION

A review of the literature indicates that, historically, the CNO role has been considered an important leadership position for hospitals in their achievement of goals. The nature of nursing's development in concert with the hospital's development as the core entity of the health care system dates as far back as Nightingale's work on the organization of hospitals and, subsequently, the organization of nurses within hospitals (Seymer 1954; Reverby 1987). As the health care system moves toward a more community-based care delivery system, the relationship of nursing services within the increasingly diffuse care delivery system must be reconsidered. Leadership in developing this future design is needed.

The literature presents a rich history of the leadership role of the CNO in hospitals. Less is known at this time about the future expectations of this position as integrated clinical services and management become more of the norm in hospitals. The study described in this book will contribute to the literature by conveying the current changes taking place in the CNO role and functions, and by exploring what might occur in the future.

Notes

1. Director of nursing became the most commonly used title for the CNO role in U.S. hospitals up until the major change by hospitals in the early 1980s to the use of corporate titles for most of their executive management staff. It remains a common title used in some community hospitals or to denote responsibility for a specific component or division of the department of nursing.

2. As an officer of ASNSA at this time, the author was personally involved in discussions with Alex McMahon that led to recognition by AHA of the CNO as a member of the institution's executive leadership team.

3

Study Approach

T he purpose of the study described in this book was to examine the role of the hospital CNO during a time of dramatic change within the health care industry. The process undertaken for this examination of change was drawn from both the literature and the author's 35 years in hospital management, nearly 25 of which were spent as a CNO. This chapter explains the study's conceptual framework and its research design.

CONCEPTUAL FRAMEWORK

To guide the search for changes in the CNO role within the context of a restructured hospital environment, a framework for analysis was developed based on the different concepts of role within organizations. In large measure, development of this framework was drawn from the work of Mintzberg (1973). Two aspects of his work, in particular, were adapted for use in the study's conceptual and analytical framework: a delineation of managerial roles and a contingency theory for managerial work.

Delineation of Managerial Roles

As discussed in chapters 1 and 2, the concept of role incorporates the idea that all positions have an attached set of organized and expected behaviors. Individuals also bring unique contributions to their role, contributing, either more or less, to the interactions of others within their group set. In organizations, particularly those that are large or complex, positions are purposely clustered or interrelated, becoming role sets or role partners in order to better achieve common goals (Newcomb, Turner, and Converse 1965). These two aspects of role, an a priori set of behaviors and placement of the role within the hospital organization, are relevant to the current changes perceived as having an effect on the CNO role within a changing health care climate.

Mintzberg's delineation of ten roles grouped into three categories also is of significance in the examination of the CNO role. Although the three role categories established by Mintzberg—interpersonal, informational, and decisional—were used in the study, the focus was only on selected roles within each category. This focus was not intended to suggest that other roles are not part of the CNO's responsibilities but, rather, that some roles, or expected behaviors, are identified more frequently with the CNO position than others.

For the purpose of developing an analysis framework for data management, the roles as identified by Mintzberg for each of his established three categories were clustered into subcategories in this study. These subcategories are linked in the following way:

- The three interpersonal roles are called the integrator role of the CNO.
- The three informational roles are referred to as the communicator role of the CNO.
- The four decisional roles are called the designer role of the CNO.

The role of leader, identified by Mintzberg as one of the interpersonal roles, transcends all other roles and becomes an expectation within all roles. To integrate, communicate, or design systems effectively, one must do so as a leader. For the purpose of this study, the role subcategories are understood as follows.

Integrator Role   The integrator role helps unite into a common core what otherwise might be disparate organizational components. Through this blending, fragmentation is avoided and a sense of community and common goals is more likely to be achieved (Lawrence and Lorsch 1969; McClure 1989). Liaison leadership, as discussed by Mintzberg (1973, 1989), is a requirement in building the web of relationships necessary for integration and in helping the organization unite with its environment. Also inherent to this role are the important functions of coordination and interpretation.

Communicator Role   The communicator role is strongly related to the integrator as a means for consensus development and goal achievement. Symbolic interaction is an inherent part of the communicator role in highly specialized organizations such as the hospital. Understanding the role of the other is needed for consensus building, which occurs primarily through a process of continuous interaction and exchange of thought. In hospitals, this becomes crucial, for each of the multiple specialists, including nursing, tends to define situations from its own discipline, training, or experience, making consensus more difficult (Christman and Counte 1981).

At the core of the communicator role is the dissemination of information. This is a two-way process that depends on having access to essential internal information. Sending and receiving information in a timely and appropriate manner throughout multiple organizational relationships is a key role expectation of the CNO. Values and organizational direction are transmitted through this important role (Mintzberg 1973).

Designer Role As a designer of the organization, the CNO seeks continuous improvement through the facilitation and design of patient care systems (AONE 1995). The set of roles encompassed in this category relate to the involvement of managers in organizational, strategic, and operational decision-making activities within their area of responsibility and beyond (Mintzberg 1973). Thus, development of an environment for clinical practice and establishment of a vision and direction that lead to high-quality patient care are part of the CNO's designer role.

Contingency Theory for Managerial Work

The framework for examining work variables, developed by Mintzberg (1973) in his now-classic study of managers, indicates that the work of a manager at any particular time is influenced by four sets of variables: the environment, the job itself, the person in the job, and situational variables of the job that may be of a temporary nature. These variables influence the role requirements as well as the characteristics of the manager's work and help account for both the similarities of the work and the individual differences that may be found. This framework was considered a useful approach in examining basic job characteristics of the CNO in hospitals and how these characteristics are influenced by these variables, affecting the CNO's role in a particular hospital.

In the study, environment and situational variables were considered major contextual influencers. Environment was regarded primarily from the view of the influence of external factors on the hospital—that is, financial changes, managed care, and competition—as well as the hospital's history and organizational characteristics. Situational variables were considered primarily those that were part of the change/stability cycle of the hospital, and include organizational restructuring and work redesign efforts. And, just as Mintzberg described, job variables relate to the organizational placement of the CNO position and the way the functional area of nursing within the organization is defined or recognized. Finally, this framework includes variables associated more specifically with the person in the role of CNO, including tenure in the job, personal style, and personality, as well as values held.

This framework for the analysis of nursing management and CNO role change was used to respond to the four study questions presented below. Figure 3-1 displays schematically the link of the conceptual framework to the research questions.

RESEARCH DESIGN

A qualitative research project using multiple-site case study analysis was undertaken to examine the impact of change on the CNO role in hospitals. A case study strategy was chosen to provide a greater opportunity to capture real-time events and contextual conditions during this time of fluctuation in the health care field. This strategy is supported by Eisenhardt (1989), who indicated that the case study method provides an opportunity to focus on the dynamics present in single settings. Yin's (1994) five components of a research design were followed in the development of this study.

Study Propositions

Yin (1994) indicated the need for study propositions to help point the researcher in the right direction as the case study is undertaken. The following five propositions form the basis for the study questions:

P1. The current status of the CNO in the organization reflects the response of the organization to environmental factors.

P2. Changes in the CNO role that have taken place over the past three years reflect elements of professional-bureaucratic conflict or role ambiguity. (See chapter 2.)

P3. Changes in the CNO role will provide information about the context that prompts organizational change.

P4. Changes in the CNO role have an impact on the effectiveness of nursing in the organization.

P5. Changes in the CNO role will provide useful insight into how organizations accomplish change.

Study Questions

In an attempt to provide direction for the quickly changing field, in 1995 AONE responded to the changes perceived to be taking place in nurse

FIGURE 3-1. Framework for Analysis of Nursing Management and CNO Role Changes

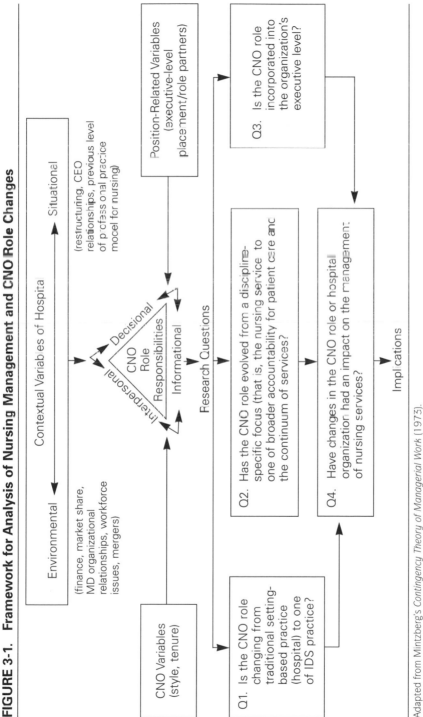

Adapted from Mintzberg's *Contingency Theory of Managerial Work* (1975).

executive practice by developing a Statement on the Role and Function of Nurses in Executive Practice. (See appendix A.) This statement was used to provide support for the four broad questions developed to guide the study. Additionally, Colloton's (1984) challenges to nurse executives, discussed in chapter 2, were used to provide another level of supporting rationale for each of these questions. This set of challenges also was used to influence the content of the interview guide. (See appendix B.)

Following are the four questions used in the study:

Q1. Is the CNO role changing from the traditional focus of setting-based practice (that is, the hospital as an autonomous health care setting) to one of an IDS practice?

Q2. Has the CNO role evolved from a discipline-specific focus (that is, the nursing service) to one of broader accountability for patient care and the continuum of services?

Q3. Is the CNO role incorporated into the organization's executive level?

Q4. Have changes in the CNO role or the hospital organization had an impact on the management of nursing services?

The relationship of the study propositions and study questions is shown in table 3-1.

Use of an Expert Panel

Because changes in the CNO role are of an evolving nature, an expert panel was used to provide content validity by confirming selected aspects of the study assumptions and the study sample. The panel was composed of four nationally prominent nurse leaders, including a CNO in an academic medical center with expanded responsibilities as COO; the executive director of a major organization representing CNOs and other nurse executives; a nurse leader who has held various key positions, including

TABLE 3-1. Relationship of Propositions and Study Questions

Proposition	Q1	Q2	Q3	Q4
1	X		X	X
2	X	X	X	X
3	X		X	X
4		X		X
5			X	X

directorship of a recently completed, funded project on change in hospital nursing; and an internationally recognized educator in nursing management and administration. These individuals were contacted first by mail and then by phone asking for their participation, and each replied affirmatively. The process of sharing information and gaining confirmation was achieved via group phone conference, fax, E-mail, and regular mail.

The expert panel members were asked to confirm the validity of the emerging patterns of CNO role change discussed in table 1-3 in chapter 1. Confirmation also was sought on the organizational and professional components of the CNO role responsibilities (table 1-2), also described in chapter 1. Finally, the study sample selection process was presented to this panel to validate the author's thinking on the priority or relevance of the criteria that should be used for the selection of study sites in this fast-changing health care environment.

Study Sample

One major challenge of the study was how to select the appropriate hospitals to serve as study sites. There are many ways to look at the changes that form the focus of this study. One way was to ask the members of the expert panel to respond to the question: Which of the following considerations is the most relevant in the selection of hospital sites to be visited and studied?

- Those hospitals that can provide an example of each of the patterns of CNO role change presumed to be occurring?
- Those hospitals that are known for having already restructured or undertaken work redesign?
- Those hospitals that have both restructured and developed IDSs?
- Those hospitals that represent one type of hospital (all academic teaching hospitals or all community hospitals)?

In the end, organizational restructuring was chosen as the framework for study site selection. Further, it was decided that the overriding consideration in selecting study sites should be those organizations that currently are influencing the field. Many different examples of hospital restructuring and work redesign exist, but system integration is a known, and considered a very likely, organizational design for the future. Thus, it was judged the most representative model for the study.

A managed care environment was regarded to be an essential consideration in determining study sites. Important also was the belief that the study sites should be those that have gained credibility in the field for their leadership or that are considered to be organizations that can be trusted to be responsible and responsive in a turbulent environment. And, finally, the sites studied should be those from which one might expect to have findings that are generalizable.

The expert panel was unanimous in its selection of three IDSs that are best known for their recent changes and thought to be in the vanguard of the changes anticipated to occur in the rest of the country. Each of these health systems was listed recently as being among the ten largest secular and not-for-profit health care systems as measured by staffed acute care beds (Greene and Lutz 1996).

Because the study sought to examine organizational change as it is affecting the CNO position in hospitals, the CEO of each IDS was asked to allow the flagship hospital of his or her IDS to serve as the study setting.[1] Interviews with each hospital's CNO and CEO were expected to provide any information that might be associated with CNO role change and the larger or parent system organization.

All three participating hospitals are located in an urban area in three different states. Also, the hospitals represent organizations of long standing, although one site is a newly merged hospital organization combining two well-known and long-standing hospitals in the same community. Table 3-2 provides a profile of the participating study hospitals. To preserve anonymity, the hospitals were identified in the study as Hospital Red, White, and Blue. Other, potentially identifying information was removed from the interviews and documents related to the hospitals and the identities of the CEO or the CNO.

Contact with each CEO was first made by letter (appendix C) and then followed up with a phone conversation to confirm both his or her willingness to participate in the study and the name of the hospital CNO. A similar letter then was sent to the CNO (appendix D), who remained the primary contact for establishing the interview schedule and providing demographic and other resource material on the hospital and the IDS.

Study Limitations

As mentioned above, the flagship hospitals of three IDSs were chosen because they were considered to be at the forefront of change. Although the systems selected are regarded as representative of what is likely to occur for many health organizations in the future, many other hospitals in the United States currently are organized within an IDS. Thus, the findings of this study are limited in that the case studies provide information only about one segment of the health care system. Certainly, restructuring and work redesign efforts are occurring even without the hospital being involved in a large IDS. It can only be presumed that changes similar to those identified in the three study hospitals are taking place

TABLE 3-2. Profiles of the Three Study Sites

Hospital	Red	White	Blue
Location	Urban	Urban	Urban
Type	Not-for-profit academic medical center	Not-for-profit teaching	Not-for-profit multispecialist teaching
Bed size:			
No. licensed	1,737	926	903
No. staffed	1,223	612	656
Total hospital FTEs (without residents and follows)	6,677	3,343	2,792
No. residents and fellows	680	40	571
Percentage of hospital revenue contracted managed care (excludes non-HMO Medicare)	26	30	30
Cost/adjusted discharge	$8,350	$8,217	$6,400

throughout the health care field. Speculation as to how the findings from the study sample might apply to the various types of hospitals and health care systems can occur, but definitive conclusions cannot be made.

Some might consider a further limitation to be the author's background as a CNO. However, her knowledge of the field provided the opportunity to immediately connect with those participating in the interviews, an advantage because of the limited time that could be spent at each of the sites.

In the early 1980s, the author served as president of AONE, which enabled her to become identified nationally as a leader in support of enhancing the CNO role on the hospital's executive leadership team. Although every attempt was made to enter each of the study fields objectively and to remain unbiased throughout the process, it is conceivable that the author's career as a CNO and experience with AONE has had an influence on the conclusions drawn from the study data.

Finally, although the author had been acquainted with some of the CNO and CEO participants prior to the time of the study, her contact with them had been episodic and related solely to professional meetings and activities. The responses of those interviewed did not appear to be affected as a result of these prior contacts, although, unquestionably, access to the study settings was made easier as a result of them.

DATA COLLECTION

As mentioned earlier, the research design used in this study provided the greatest leeway for a focused examination of organizational change as viewed through two primary study participants at each site: the hospital CNO and the hospital CEO. The CNO is the primary unit of analysis in the study with the CEO an important secondary source of analysis because of the nature of their employment relationship and the presumed impact of CEO decisions on the organization on the CNO role.

The measures used to examine the CNO role in the hospital were broadened to include individuals other than the CEO and the CNO so as to have more than just one level of the organization reporting the impact of the changes. Thus, nurse managers or others selected by the CNO were invited to participate in the interview process. In this way, a multiple-level analysis was incorporated into the research design, satisfying one of the criteria for an embedded case study design (Yin 1994). Subunits of analysis were incorporated within the semistructured interview guide and related to corresponding changes within the organization—for example, changes in leadership or budget—and their effect on the function and role relationships of the CNO.

In all three case studies, evidence was collected from multiple sources. The first and principal source of data collection was the interview. The second source, direct observation, was limited to the time allocated for the on-site visits made for the purpose of interviewing. The third source of evidence consisted of documents such as job descriptions, résumés, organizational charts, and brochures and other written material, as well as individual and institutional demographic information provided by the CNO. These three sources of evidence are included in Yin's discussion of six sources of evidence that can be used in case study analysis. A flowchart of this research design is provided in figure 3-2.

Triangulation through the use of multiple sources of evidence is highly recommended in case study analysis because of the broad range of issues usually encountered. Convergence of data from these multiple sources of evidence was carried out as Yin (1994) strongly recommends for corroborating phenomena encountered.

Throughout the process of data collection, an attempt was made to stay focused on gathering information on the facts surrounding the changes as well as on the interviewees' perceptions and opinions of those changes (Yin 1994). By doing so, the experiences of those directly

FIGURE 3-2. Research Design: Analysis of CNO Role Change

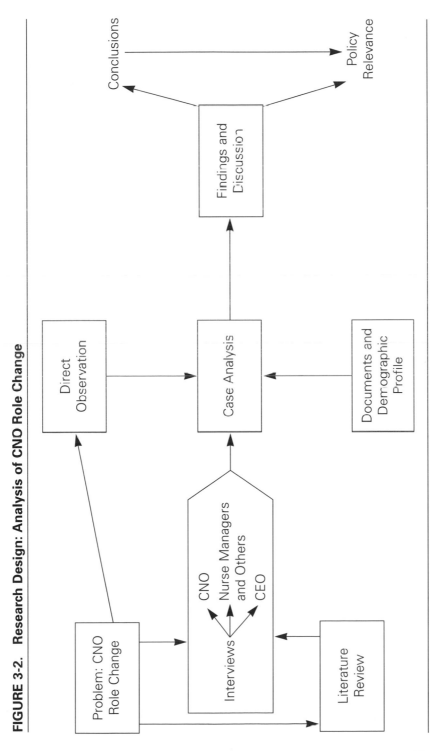

43

involved in the assumed change were expected to be captured and their significance better understood (Seidman 1991).

Interviews

On-site interviewing was conducted in June 1996 at each of the participating hospitals. The interviews were audiotaped with the permission of the people involved using a focused, open-ended discussion procedure. A semistructured interview guide (appendix B) was developed to help keep on track and yet still capture the relevant, but more global issues of organizational change that had occurred at the study site.

The interview schedule was established by the CNO. As previously indicated, she was asked to include at least three to four nurse managers in the schedule and, at her discretion, anyone else she considered helpful to the purpose of the study. An abstract of the study was provided to both the CNO and the CEO in advance of the site visit.

In total, $36\frac{1}{2}$ hours of audiotaped interviews were collected and then transcribed in their entirety by someone other than the interviewer. Each interview lasted $1\frac{1}{2}$ to 2 hours and was conducted by the author. The CEOs and CNOs were interviewed individually. Other interviews were conducted either individually or in a group. An overview of the interview schedule is displayed in table 3-3.

Direct Observation

All the interviews were conducted on site (that is, at each of the participating hospitals), generally in either a conference room or an office. In two of the hospitals, the CNOs voluntarily scheduled two interviews, one in the office during normal work hours and the other as a follow-up during the dinner hour. In the one hospital whose CNO arranged only

TABLE 3-3.   Interview Overview, by Study Site

Hospital	Red	White	Blue	Total
No. of scheduled interviews:				23
Individuals	4	9	3	
Groups	3	2	2	
Total no. of participants	32	16	16	64
No. of hours of taped interviews	11	17	8.5	36.5

one interview, the dinner hour was scheduled so as to allow the previous CNO to participate.

Although limited, the on-site interviews provided an opportunity for direct observation of the CNO, the CEO, and the nurse manager respondents in their natural work environment. Field notes from these direct observations were constructed as applicable and followed the general content of the interview guide.

Documents

Prior to visiting the sites under study, information was sought that would provide a profile of each organization, CEO, and CNO participating in the study. For example, each organization was asked to provide its organizational chart and the CNO job description—one version that was current and one that represented the organization three to five years earlier. Other relevant documents relating to the organization, new program development, or budget and staffing were sought during and after the on site visit. In each hospital, additional written information was received. The reason for gathering documentation was to build corroborating sources of evidence as described earlier.

DATA ANALYSIS

The interviews conducted in the three organizations yielded sufficient information to allow for rich content analysis from each site and to reveal common themes both within and across sites. The conceptual framework discussed earlier guided the discovery of themes and patterns, and served as an overall framework for categorizing and analyzing the data gathered from the interviews. Although these a priori categories were used in the analysis process, as suggested by Strauss and Corbin (1990), they did not limit the possibility of additional insights coming from the transcribed interviews or other documents examined.

The preliminary phase of the analysis consisted of reviewing the field notes taken and listening to selected portions of the interview tapes to either verify the written transcription or clarify the tone and inflection of the participant's voice so as to confirm the meaning intended. Throughout this phase, a coding scheme using the conceptual foundation set forth for this study was implemented. A separate file was created for each setting and transcript, and the analysis of each setting was completed before moving on to the next. Each transcript was reviewed at least three times, always returning to the audiotapes for clarification as needed. One postinterview phone conference was held with each CNO for the purpose of either clarifying areas about the organization that were vague, requesting further demographic information, or learning whether pending restructuring or redesign efforts were implemented.

Initially, areas of the transcripts that were of particular interest were identified, and on a second reading were confirmed as such and coded. The original four study questions permeated the process, as did the search for evidence of role functioning of the CNO in the three categories and subcategories described earlier: interpersonal (especially the roles of integrator and liaison leader), informational (both directions), and decisional (particularly related to the design of a patient care delivery system). Categorizing patterns and themes continued for the individual case studies using an analysis outline that served as a blueprint for grouping the findings. Each site was studied separately in order to allow the characteristics of that site to emerge (Eisenhardt 1989; Schensul and Schensul 1990).

Once the within-site analysis was completed, generalization across all three cases could be accomplished. Common patterns and themes were identified first from each site individually; then they were coded and used to identify common patterns and themes emerging from all study sites. These were then used to present the overall findings and the discussion presented in chapter 7. These procedures are intended to satisfy, in part, Yin's (1994) fourth and fifth components of case study research design.

It was not the author's intent to do a comparative analysis of the three study sites but, rather, to seek patterns and themes related to organizational change as demonstrated in the changing role of the CNO within the organization. The following three chapters are case studies of the three sites used in this study and focus on each site's particular characteristics.

Notes

1. For purposes of this study, *flagship hospital* is defined as the largest of the system's acute care hospitals that also engages in the teaching activities of medical students or postgraduate residency training.

4

Red Hospital Case Study

INTRODUCTION

Red Hospital is a large academic medical center located in a sizable city. It is the flagship hospital of a relatively newly formed IDS.

Demographics and Features

The IDS that Red Hospital belongs to consists of 13 hospitals and 6 nursing homes, and has alliances with numerous health care organizations throughout the region. The system employs more than 23,000 people and boasts a medical staff membership of nearly 4,500 physicians. Multiple outpatient facilities are associated with the system, including clinics, urgent care centers, and rehabilitation centers.

Some years earlier, the city had two very prominent hospitals—North Hospital and South Hospital. Both hospitals were known for their contributions to health care, having spent years developing competitive approaches to services in the community. Moreover, both had a strong and proud institutional culture related to patient care and academic medicine. In 1992 the decision was made to merge the two hospitals into a single corporation, which took place four years later. These two former competitors now were expected to integrate services and collaborate as one. Their medical staffs also were merged into one staff for the now major tertiary hospital of the health system. The merger was expected to eliminate excess capacity from the system.

However, complicating the issues of hospital integration was the simultaneous expansion of the newly formed and still developing IDS. Two health systems and another major hospital were added to the system within the next two years, each of which had a long history of independence, competition, and deeply rooted tradition and culture embedded in its individual identity. Motivation for these changes is attributed to health industry market trends, including managed care, the pressure for consolidation once one system had developed, and, of course, the search for economies of scale and the opportunity to increase competitive advantage. Although most of those involved understood the reasons for the changes, the magnitude of change yet to be encountered was overwhelming.

Environmental Context

More than 40 hospitals, including two major teaching medical centers, 14 HMOs, 17 PPOs, and numerous community health services and related health service businesses, reside in the region in which Red Hospital is located (Singer 1996). At a 43 percent penetration level, PPO membership has shown a slight increase over the previous year compared to the 25 percent penetration level for HMOs, which represents stability in that market for the same time period. The area's uninsured is estimated at 14 percent of the total population (Interstudy Competitive Edge 1996; Singer 1996).

Today, the influence of the several large IDSs located in the area is being threatened by the growing number of national managed care organizations (MCOs) moving in. Merging and downsizing have begun, and the IDSs are being forced to quicken the speed of their cost-cutting in order to compete effectively. Opportunity for success in these efforts is considered possible, given that, until recently, no real reduction in hospital capacity or consolidation of providers and systems had taken place (Ginsburg 1996).

Health care reform was debated in one legislative session in 1993 and 1994, hardly sufficient time to persuade market players that reform was an important policy direction (Katz and Thompson 1996). In mid-1995, the state began to implement Medicaid managed care and recently moved nearly all state employees into managed care plans (Katz and Thompson 1996).

Restructuring Efforts

In large measure, Red Hospital's restructuring efforts relate to the need to integrate duplicate clinical services and functions stemming from the merger described above. The decision to use clinical service lines as the organizational design for the merged hospital is significant in this case study.[1] This approach to the organization of clinical services was initially led by the chairman of the board of directors of what had been the larger of the two hospitals. As a successful businessman, he urged the concept of product line to be brought to the hospital because it had been so effective in business. However, the actual design of the clinical service lines was heavily influenced by the medical school and corresponds to the way its departments are divided. The concept of clinical service lines is an important influencer in the development of the structure of the merged organizations and is viewed as an instrument for implementing change at this hospital.

With a clinical service line or product line approach, an identifiable nursing department no longer exists at the hospital. Nor has the nursing department been redesigned to become a more inclusive patient care services department, as has occurred recently in some other hospitals. Nursing services are dispersed throughout the organization without central line administration or leadership except for some very specific, professionally required activities that remain part of the CNO's redesigned role responsibility. Both clinical nursing staff and nursing management staff report in various ways depending on the clinical service line they work within. Nursing is the only discipline that has not retained a departmental identity in the process of organizational structural change, and no one was able to explain why this was so. Other disciplines, such as social service and rehabilitation services, have remained with a professional department identity, even though their services also have been decentralized within the various clinical service lines.

The traditional position of nursing clinical director was changed to one called service line director, which encompasses strategic, planning, and operations responsibility. One service line director described it as being like the CEO of one's own company. Because the service lines are limited to the merged hospital, the service line directors generally do not have responsibility across the larger system. However, for some specialties, obstetrics in particular, linkages have formed, and a system-level service line executive officer is responsible for overall planning. Although it is not a requirement that the service line director position be filled by a nurse, most were. It was stated that this was the desire of the medical clinical chiefs who preferred working with nurses in those roles. However, the service line directors reported that their positions again are in flux and that they do not know what to expect in the future. A fuller description of the impact of clinical service lines on organizational structure is presented later in this case analysis.

CHANGE AT RED HOSPITAL

Surprise, just short of shock, was the response of the local community when the alliance between North Hospital and South Hospital was announced in 1992. However, no one was more surprised than the current CNO of the now-combined hospital, herein referred to as Red Hospital. The CNO was on vacation when she received the news by phone from a colleague who, like her at that time, was a member of North Hospital's senior management team. She was not alone in her astonishment, for the plans to merge the two hospitals had taken place behind the scenes and had excluded most of senior management until such time that the announcement was imminent. Although the official date of consolidation was January 1996, the events following the 1992 announcement are important in understanding the transitions now ongoing in consolidating the two hospitals.

It seemed that neither hospital CNO was involved in the decision that led to the merger, even though it was clear that a merger would have a substantial impact on the organization of nursing services. A clinical service line organization model was brought to Red Hospital, calling for a highly decentralized management structure for clinical operations, especially for the nursing service component. In fact, the notion of product line was not completely foreign to the premerger South Hospital staff. In 1990 South Hospital already had begun to reorganize along the concept of a service line organization. The CNO considered this to have been successful, primarily because the senior managers of all the service lines had a clinical background, mostly in nursing.

Evolution of the Two CNO Positions into One

When the announcement of the merger was first made, each hospital had its own CNO and senior management staff. Although change had been occurring in both roles in response to normal market and environmental forces, it was the need to think about how to integrate services that first brought the CNOs together. They began by planning ways to integrate clinical practice, using staff vacancies to create new roles in one organization and merged roles in the other. Ultimately, the process included consolidation of the two CNO roles into one at Red Hospital, creating a substantial change in that role's function.

Premerger CNO Position Functions   The South Hospital CNO had been in her position nearly 10 years at the time of the merger. Structurally, there were major differences in the way the two hospitals were organized. North Hospital had the traditional structure of a department of nursing services, whereas South Hospital was organized more around product lines with multiple vice presidents, each of whom assumed overall accountability for a single line. The incumbent CNO at South Hospital had responsibility for a service line as well as for nursing leadership across the organization. This structure was the result of many changes occurring over a four- to five-year period, beginning in 1990.

Regardless of the structural differences in their roles, however, both CNOs described their premerger work with nursing in similar ways. Essentially, both focused on the development of nursing practice and the organizational structure to support that practice. Decentralizing decision making, developing or designing the practice model, establishing appropriate staffing levels and ratios, determining salary structures, and performing other essential infrastructure work in support of nursing practice were all important functions. Both CNOs spent time with nurse managers and directors as they developed the care delivery model. Providing direction for the future and serving as a major interface for clinical nursing staff with the larger organization also were essential elements of both roles.

At South Hospital, a critical change in the CNO's role occurred when she took on responsibility for the revenue side of program management as well as the expense side. Admittedly, as a member of the senior management team, she had been involved in this before but not in such a formal, accountable way. The merger increased her level of business accountability as well as operational accountability for many programs. This placed her in direct working relationships with the medical clinical chiefs and their division chiefs, differently than before becoming more involved now in new business development activities for clinical programs and accepting responsibility for the financial outcomes. Nursing was decentralized, with 10 nursing directors who reported to her assuming operational responsibility. Her own performance evaluation at the end of the year, she indicated, was not based on the effectiveness of the nursing services but, rather, on how well her business plans did.

At the time of the interview, this nurse was no longer in the CNO position but was, instead, one of two interim administrators at Red Hospital. The other interim administrator was a former member of the senior management team at North Hospital and not a clinician. The presidents of the merged hospitals no longer were with the organization, and a search was under way for a president for Red Hospital. Transitional leadership was in place, not only for the two interim administrator positions but also for the medical director and several other senior management positions.

For 20 years before the merger, the current CNO of Red Hospital had held line responsibility at North Hospital for all inpatient nursing units, the emergency department, the clinics, and the school of nursing. As an integral part of the executive management team, she reported directly to the hospital's president and CEO. Her description of her work before 1992 suggests that the organization had had great stability for most of her tenure. The organizational structure was relatively small; four or five individuals comprised senior management. Their working relationships were described as close and family oriented. In addition to being a fully participating member of the senior administration, prior to the merger, this CNO had been a nonvoting member of the

Medical Executive Committee (MEC) and occasionally attended board meetings. There was a board committee on nursing that was very influential. She described her feelings about her working relationships as follows: "So, I've led sort of a wonderful life here. It's been great, great freedom and support. Low and behold, along came the old merger. The affiliation. I'll never forget spring of 1992."

Initially, the affiliation retained two separate CNOs, each occupying her former position. However, when change began in the CNO role of North Hospital, it was quick and dramatic. It was associated with decisions about the overall organization and administration of clinical service lines, and it was traumatic for the incumbent: "So how has my role changed? I think there was one traumatic moment when I was sort of stripped of all my line of authority."

As mentioned earlier, the former hospital presidents appear to have followed the lead of the chairman of the board and mandated that the evolving merged hospital organizational structure be developed along clinical service lines and that the ancillary and support services be integrated. Although this happened prior to the official merger, the vice presidents of both hospitals met several times and began dividing up areas of responsibilities. In the end, it seemed that there was one more vice president than was needed for operational responsibilities.

CNO Role Redesigned   Initially what emerged was a CNO staff role for North Hospital only. After nearly 25 years of major line operations responsibilities, this CNO was asked to move into a staff role with very limited day-to-day operational responsibility. In her interview, she said that she was unclear on how the decision was made because she was part of the group of vice presidents who put forth the structure, but she also indicated that at the time she had a feeling she was being put to one side.

It was the CNO from South Hospital who provided an opportunity for the newly designed staff CNO position to be more involved by suggesting that an integration of some aspects of nursing practice begin even before the actual hospital merger and that the new staff CNO role for North Hospital be the one to assume that responsibility. Two CNO positions continued on each hospital campus until the official merger occurred.

As a staff position, the CNO role now has been incorporated across the two hospitals, with the CNO from North Hospital retaining that designation. She also has retained a title of vice president (for clinical support services/CNO). As indicated previously, the former CNO of South Hospital was serving as an interim administrator at the time of the interviews for this study. Reporting to her are two other vice president roles, both currently held by nurses. Together, they assume the major responsibility for clinical operations in Red Hospital, and the clinical service line directors report to them.

The incumbent CNO believes that her longevity and previous respect in the organization led to her remaining in the staff CNO position.

Moreover, she admitted that her decision to remain in the position as it was redesigned was influenced by the stage of her career. As she was contemplating retirement in a couple of years, she made no attempt to design the job differently or to negotiate for more operating responsibilities. Although understandable, this does point out how personal choices of incumbents can influence organizational design.

The changes in the calendar of the CNO have been remarkable, reflecting her staff role rather than any operational responsibilities she still has. She continues to attend weekly executive staff meetings, which are basically information-sharing sessions on financial, quality, and other administrative issues. She holds a combined meeting with her direct reports and those of another vice president, who also is a nurse. They share this meeting because her group is small, and it is easier to have the groups meet together.

The CNO indicated that she is not as busy as she once was because she no longer has a nursing department to lead. In the past, she spent more of her time with the directors and nurse managers. Now that she has the time, she is often asked to assist others by taking on special projects. She considers herself purely an administrator rather than a clinical leader or manager.

She does sit on the Chief Nurse Executive Council at the health system level of the corporation. This council is one of several established at the system level to coordinate issues that are relevant to a cross-system approach. There is no official nursing position at the system level, although the former CNO of South Hospital, as interim administrator for Red Hospital, is a member of the administrative council. She indicated that the system level is very administration and physician oriented and that to include other disciplines there on a permanent basis would be "unnatural." On the other hand, the nonclinical interim administrator indicated that he has recommended that when a more permanent organizational structure is in place, there should be a place at the system level of leadership for a nurse such as his counterpart, arguing that her sensitivity to patient care and clinical issues makes her contribution different from his.

The Council of Nurse Executives coordinates issues that need to be attended to systemwide, sometimes through its work as a council and other times by bringing issues forward to the system's senior executive officers. The CNOs consider this to be a very workable and reasonable plan, but the clinical staff are not as happy about it, fearing that the issues of patient care will be overlooked in favor of the business and financial needs of the system. At the same time, nurse managers and others are unclear about the value of having a CNO at the system level if the position has no operational authority. They feel that something is missing at the system level without a CNO position but are unsure how to articulate the need. This uncertainty probably reflects the developing nature of the IDS as well as the traditional interest of clinicians that decisions affecting patient care programs be developed by, or at least with, clinicians.

LEADERSHIP DIMENSIONS AND THE CNO ROLE

Throughout the site visit and analysis of the interview data, evidence of the leadership dimensions of the CNO role was sought, particularly in those areas considered to be essential components of the conceptual foundation of organizational and professional leadership expectations— the CNO as integrator, communicator, and designer providing vision and direction for the whole. Indeed, there was little evidence that these leadership functions were being carried out, although those interviewed offered a good deal of discussion supporting the need for them within the organization. Given the lack of a central nursing department and the redesigned CNO staff role at Red Hospital, the roles of integrator, communicator, and designer for patient care delivery were deemed absent by those interviewed.

CNO as Communicator

On the one hand, the decentralization of clinical management, especially that of nursing, through the use of service line management structures is viewed as having improved the interdisciplinary work within a service line. On the other hand, however, it seems that the systems that were created are much more cumbersome to work through to achieve results. The communication hierarchy is said to have become more complicated in the absence of a central relationship with the CNO. With multiple reporting relationships now an intrinsic part of the service line structure, the CNO role has become unclear to nurse managers, who, in the past, had always known that their concerns eventually would reach the CNO and that the CNO was ultimately responsible for decisions affecting nursing and patient care. According to the nurse managers interviewed, they no longer believe they can rely on the CNO position to advocate for patient care and nursing practice in the appropriate forums: "[In the past] there was a sense of a person who truly supported professional nursing practice and who wanted to be progressive and wanted nursing to continue to evolve in really positive ways, and there's no sense of, at least I don't feel, a sense of that any longer, that there is a person with some authority who goes in fighting for nursing."

Although some might consider these comments to be discipline specific, the underlying issue relates to consistency in clinical practice standards that leads to high-quality patient care. With multiple reporting relationships, differing priorities, and leadership that may or may not be clinically grounded, nurse managers question how the organization as a whole will ensure that standards are set and met and that quality is consistent for the community served.

CNO as Integrator

The nurse managers also felt that the CNO's integrator role is missing and believed that communications are more problematic now because there is no central way to evaluate the impact of change on others. For example, because each service line has different priorities, something viewed as unimportant to one service line may be dropped even though it may be needed by another or needed to ensure consistency in patient care. Clinical nurse specialists spoke of this in particular as they attempted to ensure consistency in standards for groups of patients such as those with cardiac disease or diabetes who were hospitalized in a different service line. Changes in other departments such as pharmacy or material management were also cited as difficult to implement across the multiple service lines. In the past, the nursing department had provided a channel for helping people understand the impact of change on others and facilitated the process of change.

The change in the organizational design of clinical services to service lines has led to a substantial change in the CNO role. The interviewees pointed out that although much of the CNO's work may be invisible to many in the organization, it is incredibly important. Coordinating with other programs, performing liaison leadership activities, and establishing a common vision and helping others reach it are among the position's responsibilities. As one interviewee put it: "If it is everyone's responsibility, it becomes no one's responsibility; and for nursing, there are just too many nurses in too many parts of the organization not to have someone really focusing on common issues." In general, this statement relates to the important role of integration that nursing plays within an organization, but in particular, it points out the importance of the CNO role as integrator. At the time of the study, there was no evidence that this role had been taken on by the incumbent CNO nor that opportunities existed for her to take it on given the design of the CNO role as a staff position within the hospital.

CNO as Designer

An important function ascribed to the conventional CNO role is that of designer of the structure that supports clinical practice and promotes professional development. With an organizational structure of autonomous service line divisions and a CNO role that holds no operational authority for nursing practice or patient care outcomes, the opportunity to design systems for practice and patient care is limited within the staff CNO position. However, redesigning the care delivery system is a current project led by the former South Hospital CNO, now an interim hospital administrator. The current staff CNO of Red Hospital leads one of the multidisciplinary redesign teams but otherwise is not involved with nursing staff in designing the structure for patient care. Rather, she is involved in the further development of a center for nursing research that she and the former CNO of South Hospital established prior to the merger.

IMPACT ON THE ORGANIZATION OF THE CNO ROLE CHANGE

Red Hospital is not only adapting to change in response to the health care environment but also is trying to become a new entity built on the foundation of two, previously well-established and successful institutions. At the time of the study, the official merger had taken place only six months before. The organization's top leadership was interim only and the situation of its nursing leadership unclear. The change in function of the designated CNO role is substantial and not simply an issue of a position moving from line accountability for all of nursing to staff accountability for nursing within the senior management team. The staff CNO has limited access to nursing staff except for those nurses who report directly to her (a director of nursing practice and a director of nursing systems). She has assumed administrative responsibility for a very limited number of clinical areas, not because she is the CNO but, rather, because she (1) has had a lot of experience in the organization, (2) has had a very light workload compared to others, and (3) has adopted the attitude that she would "help out," or as she puts it: "Give me whatever you need to get done, [and] I can sort of do it."

Loss of Influence in the Organization

The loss of the CNO's organizational influence was evident in many ways. The CNO herself described her role as follows: "I'm unempowered. I'm now a staff person up here . . . and all I can sort of do is influence by influence." However, she found this to be somewhat acceptable because after so many years with one of the hospitals, she remained loyal and wanted the organization to have whatever it felt was best. Her concern was primarily for the past investment that had produced a good patient care delivery system, and she did not want that to be lost. Her perspective was altruistic: "I have no self-interest. It doesn't matter to me—titles, role, autonomy, or authority—I could give it up. I just want to be what is good for that place."

An important example of this change in influence is the relationship the CNO now has with the medical staff, a group that is quite influential in this hospital. Speaking of the change in relationship, the nonclinical interim administrator indicated that the degree of direct contact has lessened. Although the CNO still sits on committees such as the MEC, the work she does with the clinical chiefs of medicine is not the same because nursing no longer reports directly to her. If the chiefs need to work out operational issues, they go to either the clinical service line directors or the vice presidents because they do not view the CNO as having any authority over the work that needs to be done. This example and others (some of which are described later) illustrate that, except for very specific nursing issues, the CNO's involvement in planning for the future is limited. It also brings to the forefront the concept of role partners and how sensitive those relationships are in an organization.

The CNO of Red Hospital is well known by many members of the medical staff as a result of having worked with some of them for two decades and she continues those personal relationships, but she also recognizes her diminished involvement with the medical staff in terms of clinical operations and planning. When asked what she would really like to have back in her role, she said: "I think I'd like to have more influence, if that's the word. Maybe I have it now, and I just haven't learned how to get it across."

All this suggests that the lack of authority in the redesigned CNO role has had an impact on the organization in various ways. For nurse managers, the lines of authority above them are perceived to be diffuse and thus impede their ability to move forward with a sense of common direction. For the CNO, the consequences of not having line authority are a diminishing in her ability to be influential in her relationships with nurse managers and other organizational leaders.

Operational Impact of Decentralization

Those interviewed expressed a sense of loss that relates to many aspects of the important roles identified for leaders as integrators and communicators. Through their presence, interactions, and involvement with others, leaders interpret organizational dynamics and direction within and among groups, and provide comfort, particularly during times of change.

The nurse managers were intense in their descriptions of their loss at no longer meeting regularly as a group to work with the CNO and nursing directors, to share collegiality, and to communicate with each other. Even when the nurses disagreed with each other, the meetings had always made them feel centrally focused and directed. At best, this loss of a central forum for nursing managers has led to diminished cohesiveness; at worst, it has weakened their morale, direction, and ability to motivate staff.

The nurse managers are not the only ones in the organization affected by the change in the CNO role. Clinical nurse specialists also spoke of the impact on their positions of the changes in the CNO role and the design of service line divisions. They felt themselves to be less visible to the organization because they report in "scattered" ways throughout. Thus, they are less likely to be viewed as a resource outside a particular service line. There is an absence of a common vision and direction for these advanced practice nurses, who generally provide an organization with a needed level of expertise in clinical standard setting and monitoring. As they individually try to approach the multiple service line divisions, they are met with inconsistency, depending on the current agenda and service line priorities. They describe the process of trying to get people to see problems across the hospital system as one that requires them to "jump through many hoops" because each service line acts independently of the others. It is difficult to bring a central focus to an issue. To do so requires that they deal with more, rather than fewer, organizational layers because each service line must be approached individually.

Finally, attendees at a combined department meeting voiced a great deal of frustration about the loss of the CNO as someone who could facilitate and help integrate the care delivery system needs with the issues of the larger organization. They viewed the lack of consistency around patient care goals for the organization as a critical loss for the hospital. Previously, the CNO had interacted with the board, the medical staff, and the administration. Now there is no longer a single resource at the senior level for the integration work perceived to be needed.

Change in Nursing Service Management and Administration

One result of the change to product or service line management has been a change in the reporting relationships of some nurse managers. A hierarchy of reporting relationships still exists; that is, the nurse manager reports to a clinical service line director, who reports to a vice president, who reports to a senior vice president. However, the difference is that the roles above the nurse manager are not necessarily nursing roles, and even in those situations where the incumbent is a nurse, the organizational design does require that to be so. This differs from the organizational relationships that have remained for other disciplines, all of which have retained a direct line to their own discipline even though, operationally, they might be decentralized to a service line.

The change in the nurse managers' reporting relationships and role began with development of the clinical service lines, an organizational model intended in part to improve interdisciplinary work by breaking down the potentially narrow or isolated approach of departments, now often referred to as the silo approach. According to those interviewed, however, interdisciplinary work has improved within each service line, but the service lines themselves seem to have become silos and, in some ways, more problematic. Each service line is expected to stand on its own. Thus, it has the potential to be more isolated from overall organizational goals because of a strong focus on achieving its own goals and because of the lack of a central means to communicate plans and progress. Although nursing services are present in all service lines, they no longer are matrixed to any central leadership. Consequently, nursing as the nexus for patient care in the organization has been lost.

For many of the nurse managers at Red Hospital, access to the top levels of the organization also seems to have been lost. That was one of the roles the CNO traditionally played: linking those in direct clinical care with the mission, goals, and strategic direction of the larger organization. The nurse managers now feel far less in touch with what is going on in the hospital. In her formal role, the CNO, like the clinical directors, was a crucial link in information sharing. Moreover, because the service line directors have broader administrative responsibility than they had in the past as clinical directors, now they too are further removed from the nurse manager and have no formal relationship with the CNO. Nurse managers feel a tremendous increase in their workload, but a loss of support. One described the situation as "flying by the seat of your pants."

However, nurse managers did report enjoying the new skills they have acquired as a result of the changes in the management functions within other roles as well as their own. For the most part, they are senior experienced nurse managers and many probably were ready for new challenges. But they agreed that this has come at a heavy price. They became very intense as they described the impact the changes have had on their relationship with clinical nursing staff. There is a difference, according to those interviewed.

Clinical Staff–Administrative Relationships

The nurse managers interviewed indicated that staff morale at Red Hospital is low. This observation was supported by both the current CNO and the interim nonclinical administrator. Nurse managers suggested that the fragmentation of patient care and the lack of direction for the clinical staff play a significant part in the diminished morale. As their own roles as managers have changed, and just as they themselves feel the loss of central communication and direction, so do their staff. They believe this is made more difficult because they are increasingly removed from the clinical workplace and thus provide less direction and support to staff. One nurse manager described the change as follows: "It's fragmented care and low morale. I think if we are all struggling, they're not getting their sense of direction from us either. They can pick up on it in a minute, and here we keep telling them: 'Don't lose sight of the patient, the patient is most important.' And they are like, 'You've lost sight of the patient, you're not here to help me as much as you used to be, or you're not providing the direction I need.'"

The impact on the clinical nursing staff of the CNO's loss of influence in the organization also was described by the nurse managers. They spoke of the "trickle-down effect" and their concern that hospital decision makers would no longer know of the work of clinicians because no one is advocating for that in the right decision-making places. This is complicated by the number of changes that have happened at senior management levels and the interim nature of administration. One nurse indicated that in a single year she has had to report to five different managers, a very frustrating work situation.

The nurse managers felt that reporting to nonclinical managers was akin to doing double work because they had to explain every aspect of their jobs to a person who is not clinically grounded. Thus, their work becomes harder and more frustrating. When they had a CNO to whom they operationally related, communication was better, information was more easily disseminated, and they felt less fragmentation.

However, there is a Department of Nursing Practice that is responsible to the CNO. In this context, *nursing practice* is defined by administrative activities or tasks that are needed across all parts of the organization. It is project oriented: data generation for quality improvement efforts, JCAHO program mandate efforts, and license renewal and review are a few of this department's activities.

Regular, formal nursing management meetings no longer exist. Rather, decentralized councils with representation is the structure in place, which the nurses did not consider to be especially useful. This is particularly so because one person is not allowed to be substituted for another at meetings. As a result, the nurse managers feel extended far beyond what is reasonable to expect. The nurse manager's scope of responsibility has increased. For example, where the nurse managers might have had responsibility for the staff and patient care associated with a 30-bed unit, they now have 60 beds. The number of assistant nurse managers has decreased at the same time that the nurse managers' responsibilities have increased. With substitution at meetings not allowed and meetings being longer (as they seem to be since the merger), nurse managers find it difficult to retain the same relationship with clinical nursing staff they once had.

Change to a Clinical Service Line Approach

During an interview with the nonclinical interim hospital administrator, interesting insights emerged about the role that nursing plays at Red Hospital. The following discussion with the nonclinical interim administrator relates to the change in nursing from a departmental approach in the organizational structure to a clinical service line approach.

> ADMINISTRATOR: It's much harder, I think, to have a cohesive nursing staff with the organization structure that we have because they all have a series of different leaders, with different expectations, and who only unite at the very top. Your manager may have a different communication skill, expectation, organization structure, and so it's harder to bring the cultural change divided up this way.
> INTERVIEWER: How important is it to have a cohesive nursing group?
> ADMINISTRATOR: I think it's the only way. In the environment that we are in now, where people are frequently pooled and moved and asked to cover different areas, that's a fundamental cultural change, I think.

This discussion pointed out the difficulty that organizations face when there is no common vision or direction and also the potential for fragmentation when cultural cohesiveness, especially in nursing, is gone. This administrator indicated that it is the patient who is at risk: "They don't know about the other things swirling around you. . . . The patient's expectation is that if they go from medicine or cardiology or surgery that they are going to have the same kind [of care]. All consistent care and their expectations don't change just because of the change in nursing divisions."

It is interesting that the patient satisfaction quality scores between the two hospitals are vastly different and that the current CNO, who had been CNO in the hospital that had the higher scores premerger, has been asked to help identify what made that difference and how to spread it across the merged organization. It is curious, however, that she has been given the job of figuring out how to raise these scores, but to do so through process work without having any central influence on operations. Once again, the nonclinical interim administrator was able to shed some light on the difficult job the CNO may have in accomplishing this, given the organizational structure. When asked if he would change the CNO role in any way, he responded:

> I would reflect back to the comment I made earlier that I am concerned that because of the fragmentation that we have, how difficult it is going to be to change the nursing culture. So if I were to make the change, and I am not sure what the change would be, it would be

somehow to have a greater penetration of the consistent nursing management message to go forward across that culture. . . . I think I would like to see a strong move, organizational structure there somehow, where nursing could feel more comfortable about its own continuity.

This administrator stated his belief that nursing was the major focus of patient care interaction and that both physician and patient satisfaction were influenced more by nursing than by any other role in the organization. Nursing, he said, was on everybody's radar screen right now because nurses are in such a vulnerable position with the organizational changes taking place and because of their impact on patient care. Again, nursing as the important nexus of patient care is his focus. He extends the impact of the nursing role to the hospital's academic mission by describing the central role that nurses play in the training of medical residents.

Patient satisfaction scores were reported to be worse, as were the employee attitude survey scores. The nurse managers interviewed indicated that patient comments in general are more negative than in the past. They discussed how they and other nurses fear a loss in patient care quality. They perceive an emphasis on cost-cutting without a like emphasis on preserving quality, and they would like to learn how to achieve a balance between the two. These discussions also exposed the manager role conflict. The managers' workload has increased in a way that they perceive removes them from their important role in developing clinical nursing staff, setting the standards for good clinical care, and helping staff reach these standards. There are fewer of them than in the past, and they are stretched not only by the number of units they are responsible for and the number of FTEs they manage, but also by the increased workload associated with decentralized meetings that take them away from staff. When there was a central department of nursing, the CNO and her direct reports were more actively involved in the meetings and planning processes now in place. The dilemma, of course, is that the expertise of the on-line manager and clinical leader is needed just as much in these planning meetings for patient care programs as it is by clinical nursing staff to help them achieve excellence in their patient care activities. One questions whether either would be less important if the structure were returned to a central nursing department. The ultimate question, of course, is the impact these changes will have on the quality of patient care in the future.

CONCLUDING REMARKS

Red Hospital is undergoing a great deal of change within a set of complex circumstances. Restructuring the care delivery system has been undertaken, just as it has in many other hospitals throughout the country. But many of those hospitals are not also confronting the difficult task of merging two organizations that, until recently, had been strong competitors with a long history of prominence in the community and a strong organizational culture. The critical nature of culture and values within organizations was felt throughout the interviews at Red Hospital, highlighting how difficult it sometimes is to make changes in things that might otherwise seem simple. In addition, the magnitude of change expected to be accomplished was, at the time of the study interviews, led by many who were in interim positions.

There were strong feelings on the part of the clinical staff of being lost, having neither direction nor a common vision. Indeed, loss was a recurrent theme in the interviews conducted at this hospital. The loss of departmental identity was symbolized by the absence of an organizational chart for nursing services, but the absence of a central, strongly identified leader who has operational influence throughout the organization was the primary focus of loss. The importance of organizational leadership was underscored in many discussions and especially the need for nursing leadership to serve as an integrator and communicator for nurses and others throughout the organization. The absence of these functions highlighted the important role that all of nursing has served as the nexus for patient care within the organization.

Fragmentation was another theme that emerged from the interviews and often was viewed as the cause of much frustration. The former CNO of South Hospital suggested that one of Red Hospital's strengths is the number of nurses in senior management positions, as either vice presidents or service line directors. However, not everyone holding these positions agreed, and in one discussion the following was offered:

> All I've been able to see throughout all this chaos, and I really think that it is the fragmentation of nursing that is what is taking place, is we have multiple people represented all the way from directors to three key vice presidents in this current structure, plus really what I would consider to be the CNE [chief nurse executive] as the interim administrator. I don't think anybody really publicized or communicated the new role of the CNO for both campuses; I think it was downplayed. I think, again, there is nobody going to the tables as a single voice. . . . It is difficult to understand who is guiding the practice of nursing and all these very decentralized groups of people that are running—I think they used the word *silos;* that's a key word because that's my opinion of what is happening. I'm not sure there is good information sharing at all the different levels, what each practice is trying to accomplish from the standpoint of nursing practice.

The incumbent CNO is learning how to influence from a different organizational base—a staff administrative role. She depends on her past relationships and her own set of values and commitment to the organization in helping others make it work. She has a great interest, in particular, in developing those younger nurses who currently are in vice president positions directing selected product lines. Although this is very commendable, it is not an organizationally sanctioned part of her role and, thus, is limited.

Notes

1. The term *clinical service line* is one of many now used to describe a hospital organizational model that is built on the business model of product line management. Patient services are grouped by clinical care need or disease-related patient populations, and a strategic business unit model for managing these services is developed. In this model, the management structure for all clinical areas usually is decentralized and total authority given to the manager for the entire product or service line. Often clinical service lines replace departmental structures for some clinical services, such as nursing.

5

White Hospital Case Study

INTRODUCTION

White Hospital is an inner-city facility with 612 acute care beds. It provides all services, including a home care program, rehabilitation services, and a transitional care unit, with the exception of pediatric care. There is a commitment at both the system and hospital level to focus on community needs, especially health prevention, wellness, and primary care.

Demographics and Features

White Hospital serves as the flagship hospital for one of the two IDSs that dominate the area's managed care market. In 1996 it was one of 19 hospitals either owned or managed by its parent organization. The IDS, formed in 1994, continues to grow and currently includes nursing homes as well as other diversified health businesses, including its own health plan. Its medical professional service group includes 65 clinics; 430 physicians, most of whom are primary care doctors employed by the IDS; and nearly 6,000 MDs affiliated in some fashion with the system's health plan and hospitals. Although approximately 80 percent of the system's revenues come from managed care, less than 10 percent come from capitation.

The physician organization of the hospital is that of a large private practice model with a small number of full-time physicians. Recent state legislation focusing on slowing the rate of growth in health care costs has placed additional financial pressures on the hospital and its perceived need to change.

Environmental Context

White Hospital is located in an area considered by some to be one of the most mature managed care markets in the United States. With a combined HMO and PPO penetration of 88 percent and 34 hospitals located within the state, the potential for competition among health providers is high. However, because state law requires all HMOs to operate as nonprofits, the competition has abated somewhat. State legislation and an influential business coalition are considered the major drivers of the health care market within which White Hospital resides (Hoechst Marion Roussel 1995; Singer 1996).

The area has experienced considerable consolidation of providers and a substantial reduction in hospital capacity (Duke 1996; Ginsburg 1996). Additionally, health care reform in the state has begun with a cost-containment strategy goal of slowing the rate of growth in health care spending by at least 10 percent per year over five years (Duke 1996; Ginsburg 1996).

Restructuring Efforts

Although speed is desired in making the transformation needed to meet the financial pressures of a continuously changing environment, White Hospital also is cognizant of its organizational culture of openness with, and commitment to, its employees. The restructuring efforts now being implemented at the hospital are, in large part, the result of the work of a cross-sectional group of employees who had been taken off line for a week to work through the elements of a redesigned patient care delivery system. The design for the organization of clinical and patient care services that has evolved is an elaborate combination of services matrixed around the concept of community, which is a form of product line restructuring. Inherent within the community is the expectation that the continuum of care will be attended to.

The most significant structural changes at White Hospital are those in the nursing management role and structure, discussed in more detail later in this case analysis. Broader responsibilities have been assumed by nursing directors (now called patient care directors or clinical nurse managers), including program as well as operational management. These changes were in the early stage of implementation at the time of this study. The CNO role has expanded to include complete responsibility for selected programs in addition to retaining overall responsibility for patient care. Although some nurse managers and clinical nursing staff report to other, nonnursing vice presidents or directors, a strong central component with a stated mission and organizational design has been retained for nursing services.

CHANGE AT WHITE HOSPITAL

The process of change now under way at White Hospital is unquestionably influenced by two previous events that permeated nearly all interviews with members of this community of caregivers and administrators. One event was a citywide nurses' strike in 1984, which continues to influence decisions made a dozen years later about the organizational structure, CNO title, and the relationship of nursing services to others in the hospital.

The second event occurred in 1990, when White Hospital received one of the 20 national RWJ Foundation and PEW Charitable Trust grants for a project called Strengthening Hospital Nursing: A Project to Improve Patient Care. The hospital project funded by this grant, along with the strong leadership of a visionary CNO, provided an opportunity to begin to break away from the strong influence of the 1984 nurses' strike. The hospital began a journey of change and new direction that it considers essential for its continuing role as the flagship hospital within its IDS, which has developed over the same twelve-year period. Within this context, the newly appointed CNO, who holds the title of patient care vice president, has committed herself to redesigning the patient care delivery system within a performance-oriented framework.

Impact of CNO Transitions

At the time of the study interviews, the CNO of White Hospital had been in the position officially for only six months. She was appointed from within after having served as interim CNO for a year while the hospital conducted a nationwide search to fill the position. Previously, she had successfully served as director of a major clinical program. Her appointment followed an outside candidate's declining the job, a fact that seemed to eclipse many of the discussions at White Hospital, including those with the CNO herself. Concern had been raised during the search process as to whether the candidate would be up to the hospital's standards, considering the history of its previous CNOs, the last three of whom had achieved national professional recognition. The CEO was quite open about the nature of the search, which ultimately led to the decision that the current CNO was an equal match to the other candidates. Discussion of the CNO selection process is included here because of the importance it seemed to have for those interviewed, a point that will become clearer as the story of the change at White Hospital unfolds.

Because of the current CNO's brief tenure, and because the immediate past CNO (currently serving in the system-level corporate offices as system vice president, quality and clinical care improvement) was available for an interview, this study of the change in CNO role functioning at White Hospital spans the tenure of both CNOs.[1]

Impact of the Financial Market

According to White Hospital's CEO, the impact of the financial market on health care, especially managed care, has caused "change in this hospital to begin in every area where care is delivered." Although change is not new to this organization, the feeling now is that the speed and pressure to reduce costs have increased substantially. The CEO assesses the impact of this on nursing: "Nursing is affected strongly because [nurses] are so essential in effecting the change that physicians must make in their practices—that is, length of stay, ambulatory continuum of care, and so on. Nurses manage patient care in terms of lower length of stay. . . . [Nurses] have to help make it happen more than any other group, in my mind."

Many of those interviewed considered finances to be a major influencer for change in this organization at this time. The end of the RWJ/PEW grant came at the same time as the financial pressures increased, and both these events coincided with the appointment of the current CNO. Thus, it became essential that she take on the role of bringing efficiency to the system. Her style has been performance oriented, a style perceived to be very different from that of the previous CNO who was well liked and well respected by everyone and characterized as a woman of "vision and wisdom." One nurse leader put it this way: "We've switched from a vice president who was very global in thinking, very visionary, to one who is more performance oriented, and I think that choice was made precisely because of the financial situation." Although the nurse leader considered this a necessary direction, she alluded that this was also part of the reason others in nursing were cautious in embracing the CNO as their new leader.

Influence of the Nurses' Union

As mentioned earlier, a citywide union strike by RNs in 1984 was a touchstone event for White Hospital and created a division among staff, nursing, and others that continues to linger a dozen years later. According to one staff member, "Until all who lived through that strike turn over, the pain will never go away." It is said that every time there are contract negotiations, the wounds of the past are opened and "stories are told and retold." Decisions about organizational structure, CNO title, and other change activities have related in part to the feelings associated with that event.

Following the strike, the CNO at the time was left to stabilize and heal the nursing department, and in her attempt to accomplish this, she developed a protective posture that was perceived by some outside the department to be somewhat insular. Although she succeeded in pulling the nurses together, by the time she left, the needed bridge building with other parts of the organization still had not been accomplished. It was left to the next CNO to begin that process. Her tools were embedded in the RWJ/PEW grant that had been developed and funded under her predecessor. The new CNO endorsed the vision of the grant and used it as a tool for moving forward.

During the interviews, the immediate past CNO spoke of her work with the nurses' union, confirming that it had consumed a large part of her time. She brought to the organization interest-based bargaining, a new technique that changed the structure of union contract negotiations. This was high risk-taking behavior on her part, for everyone still remembered the experience of the strike and no one wanted to chance another one. However, her technique proved successful in more ways than one. For one thing, she succeeded in getting other members of the administrative staff to start thinking of union activity as a problem that belonged to everyone in the hospital and not just the nurse administrator.

The current CNO is trying to heal the organization from another perspective, trying to be inclusive in her administration, and taking on the perspective of all areas of patient care even though they are not necessarily within her own scope of management responsibility. It is within the context of the bitter nurses' strike of 1984—that pitted nursing against others in the organization—that the current CNO began her leadership work for the organization:

> What that did was, it pitted nursing against all others and it forever took its toll. So my point in this whole thing in coming into this role, and as I've gone out to meet with the key department heads, like pharmacy, x-ray, social services, nutrition, infrastructure, all of that is, I'm here not as a nursing person, I am here as a patient care person and how can we work together to enhance patient care. And so, it's dispelling the anxiety around nursing.

Influence of the RWJ/PEW Grant

Receiving a funded grant was and remains a very special event for White Hospital in promoting hospitalwide organizational change. The multiple initiatives developed within the grant continue to be used as a strategy to involve others in the change process. The CEO confirmed the importance of the grant "not for the money as much as the challenge and the thinking that came as a result of that." The grant provided an opportunity to realize a system view of patient care, and as a result, total quality management (TQM) became an important tool for the hospital. TQM has helped the hospital maintain a patient focus in its redesign initiatives, and the grant is considered to have been instrumental in making a difference in the integration of disciplines.

Influence of Nonnurse Administrators

Among the contextual findings of the White Hospital visit was one spoken of by nurses as an important variable in designing the organization's nonnursing administrative structure. The hospital has served as a training ground for numerous graduates of the strong local graduate program in hospital administration. Its reputation for developing administrators who are then recruited to other hospitals across the country is well established. This is a competitive process, and the number and kind of departments that report to the administrator while at White Hospital is considered an important part of developing a successful résumé. However, an unintended consequence of this may be the influence their career aspirations have on the hospital's organizational design decisions.

Developing nursing services as a single, cohesive, professional clinical department is less of a consideration for the administrative group than is the number of departments and FTEs reporting to any given administrator. Some nurses are managed outside their discipline, and although there is an attempt to differentiate nursing affairs from operational management, the sense was that, in some areas, the CNO is responsible for holding the nurses accountable for meeting practice and patient care standards without the requisite organizational authority. This issue was addressed by members of the nursing management group as well as by the present and previous CNO, and is described again later in this study.

LEADERSHIP DIMENSIONS AND THE CNO ROLE

Analysis of the White Hospital data began with a search for evidence of the conceptual foundation associated with the dimensions of organizational and professional leadership described earlier. Indicators of the CNO's functioning as an integrator, communicator, and designer were looked for as the interview transcripts were categorized and analyzed.

CNO as Integrator

The CNO's liaison work was spoken of directly by White Hospital's CEO and is clearly viewed as an important and necessary function for the hospital as a whole. It is work that he sees her spending a lot of time on and that she considers necessary in building relationships that will bring people along in their understanding of change. The CNO's functions of interpreting to nursing staff and relating to multiple stakeholders in the organization help others to integrate. She herself indicates that she works on developing strategies that will bring others close to the core work of the organization.

Affirmation of the significance of integration through liaison leadership came from many other members of the nursing management and leadership group interviewed, especially with regard to its importance in integrating and coordinating patient care. Although the CNO is not herself directly involved in the care process, helping others sort out workload issues and responsibility relationships is viewed as being organizationally essential. Also, her work with physician leadership groups was cited by many. The medical director, for example, indicated that nurse-physician collaboration is a very important element of achieving high-quality patient care and acknowledged that such care is a team effort.

CNO as Communicator

The importance of the CNO's role as a visible communicator of change was articulated by many interview participants at White Hospital, especially members of the nursing leadership group. They frequently spoke of looking to the hospital plan for the direction and vision of the future. One nurse manager stated that "one of the most important roles for her [the CNO] is to just get out with people and just listen and talk." The need for the CNO to develop strategies for interacting with clinical staff was noted frequently. The CNO herself recognized this: "I need to be visible, to be able to inspire people to feel the vision that we've created, and in so doing bring nurses and physicians together."

In the current environment of change, such interactions were viewed as being highly valued, yet it was noted that the CNO role was less involved with clinical staff now than previously. This perception may be associated with two simultaneous phenomena: (1) the newness and style of the current CNO, and (2) a sufficient change in the CNO position responsibilities leading to less direct involvement with just nursing staff. The nursing staff interviewed explained that they look to the CNO to help clinical staff feel empowered, and because of the sheer size of the nursing workforce, such empowerment becomes important to the organization in meeting its goals. Without this, they say, the potential for adversarial relationships within the organization is heightened. It was stated that one requirement of the CNO role is to remove barriers organizationally and professionally: "If practice is to be changed, then we need the leadership of the CNO to sanction that change."

And finally, the CNO's communicator role was discussed as being useful to all in the organization—that it is through this flow of information that the CNO keeps others challenged and thinking more broadly. This process leads to more information sharing, and those outside nursing begin to get to know more about the core work of patient care, thus achieving integration.

CNO as Designer

According to many interviewed, the CNO's leadership role includes providing stability for the organization through the design of a patient care system that balances the need for change with the need to preserve a foundation of known values. The CEO expressed his expectation that the CNO would take the lead on a major reorganization of care delivery. Designing systems for participation, defining boundaries, and building bridges for the future are expectations of the CNO held by some members of the nursing leadership staff. The CNO herself believes that data, a well-rounded management team, and judicious use of expert advanced practice nurses (APNs) are some of the components needed to build a system that will provide high-quality, cost-effective care.

IMPACT ON THE ORGANIZATION OF THE CNO ROLE CHANGE

Data analysis sought not only evidence of change in the CNO role but also evidence of the impact of change on the organization. The elements of change found and their subsequent impact are incorporated in the following description of the CNO role at White Hospital.

Increased Responsibilities

In the CEO's view, the role that is changing the most at White Hospital is the CNO's. He sees her increased involvement in overall administrative responsibilities and organizational leadership for program development as the major change. He indicated that having a background in nursing is a plus for this work and that the current environment of financial pressure and change calls for new skills and change in the sets of people and organizational relationships. The CNO's decision making in this organization also has taken on increased importance, according to the CEO.

In the past three to five years, much of the CNO's time was spent designing the structure for the nursing department, developing a management team, and creating change for the larger organization. Words used by members of the administrative and nursing leadership team to describe this role included "guiding," "mentoring," "facilitating," and "coaching." They viewed the CNO as a strategist, a builder, and an integrator.

The nursing department now perceives changes in the CNO role functioning, and although these are articulated by some as being positive and as continuing the work begun by the previous CNO, a tentativeness remains in their descriptions that suggests they are waiting to see what will really happen under the current CNO's leadership. In particular, the nurses are ambivalent about how they view the CNO's strong identification with the hospital's physician group. Although they are pleased that she has such a high level of respect and trust from that group, they are nevertheless somewhat concerned that such a relationship might cause the CNO to represent the physicians' needs rather than those of nursing. This concern stems from their own worry about the complexities associated with fast-moving change and the fact that this CNO has not been in her job very long. Can they trust her? Will she have sufficient influence as a new member of the organization's leadership team? These and similar questions associated with the transition from a well-known and well-respected leader to a relatively unknown one form the basis for apprehension among White Hospital's nursing management and leadership staff.

Changes in the CNO's day-to-day work include more involvement with the medical staff (including attendance at medical board meetings), which is different from the previous CNO's activities. This CNO makes specific plans to engage physicians in patient-related discussions and activities. She joins them at breakfast, brings them on rounds to visit patients, and attends their meetings. The current CNO places great emphasis on establishing good relationships with the medical staff, and the CEO confirms the importance of this for the changes that are needed in the clinical areas. But it is efficiency in care that is the CEO's ultimate priority. When asked whether he had different expectations for the chief nurse today than he did three to five years earlier, he said: "Yes, I think much greater expectation around the efficiency of care. Before cost-base reimbursement, whatever you did you got paid for, now it's even moving from there to DRGs and some of the pressure there." Essentially, he believes that the majority of the cost of the organization lies within the CNO's responsibility, and thus she must assume accountability for the efficiency of patient care.

The CEO also articulated an extension of this requirement of the CNO role, saying that it is the CNO who has the major responsibility for redesigning care delivery for the hospital. She is expected to take the lead in this area of reorganization and to present the design for care delivery to the medical staff and board as well as to everyone else. Her organizational placement as an integral member of the President's Council and other executive staff committees and activities provides her the opportunity to fulfill these expectations. Working closely with the senior management team and medical staff is the area the CEO describes as having changed the most for the current CNO. This change occurred because the CEO recognized that the CNO was really the key to operations. Thus, he expanded her responsibilities to include more program areas as well as nursing. CNO access to the President's Council began only a few years ago, so this sphere of influence opportunity is relatively new in her role at White Hospital.

CNO participation in the President's Council, the medical board, and other, similar senior-level organizational activities is meaningful to the role partners found at this level of the organization. It suggests in part that her role is considered influential and might be helpful to them in achieving their own organizational goals. Changes in other hospital committees are occurring as well, including the integration of nursing administration leadership within broader patient care committees.

According to the CNO, the chief nurse's role is no longer to look only at the service provided within the hospital. As the chief nursing leader in the flagship hospital of an IDS, she is involved in designing systems that will help follow patients across the continuum of services needed. Working with the CNOs of other systemwide facilities is part of this expanding role, and representing both nursing and the hospital at the system level of planning is beginning to consume more of her time as well. There is a nurse executive/patient care council at the corporate level of the system that she attends and takes turns at chairing.

Trying to balance her responsibilities in the hospital with commitments in the IDS has become difficult. For example, she has to prioritize attendance at multiple and overlapping meetings. Moreover, she is concerned about the perception of others that she does not care about their issues. This problem, it seems, is greater for the CNO than for others in executive leadership because they tend to have more discrete areas of responsibility.

And indeed, some nurses at White Hospital are worried that expanding the CNO's responsibilities and integrating her role to this extent may dilute the advocacy activities that clinical nursing staff seek from her to ensure that the top of the organization understands the real work of nursing in patient care. However, others see the change as useful in expanding the role they previously saw as the "spiritual leader for nursing" to a broader organizational "guardianship" role for patient care. Whatever the case, they see the CNO role as important in educating members of the larger hospital community about the impact of change on the actual experiences of patients and families in an environment that is quickly and dramatically changing.

Expanded Boundaries

The title of patient care vice president held by the current CNO began with the appointment of the previous CNO. To date, however, the scope of responsibility included in this position title has not included departmental responsibility for disciplines beyond nursing. Some operational program responsibility that includes other disciplines is being assumed by the current CNO, whereas the previous CNO held operational responsibility for nursing only. However, it was the previous CNO who, at the time of her appointment, negotiated the broader title of patient services in order to begin the process of integrating and healing the organization from the damage that was perceived to have occurred with the nursing strike of 1984.

The CEO indicated that organizational change began with this change in title. It was the beginning point of the project of redesign to be undertaken, and he felt that it was a way to establish a framework for leading patient care change: "What I had in mind was not so much the direct reporting relationships, for example that physical therapy and respiratory therapy and all those things would come under the CNO. It was more that this was the person who would oversee everything—whatever happened to the patient, which included some of those things. They didn't have to report in to her, but when we did our governance councils and all of our patient care councils, they were going to be brought around the table and be a part of this patient care team, which the CNO would lead. It was more of a team approach than a direct reporting relationship."

The CEO focused on changing the relationships of others to the CNO, and to nursing in general, not through the process of direct reporting but, rather, through the strategy of team-building councils. Again, his caution in communicating changes in relationships with nursing leadership relates, in part, to his sensitivity to the feelings of other members of the hospital organization toward nursing as a result of the strike a dozen years earlier. Evidence of this sensitivity also was identified in discussions with the CNO when speaking of the integration of other disciplines into a redesigned patient care system. When asked whether she currently managed clinical departments other than nursing, she responded: "Not at this moment in time, because back in 1984 and the strike, there is not one single person who wants nursing to manage them at all, they will not be taken and so what I will very strategically and intentionally do is work with them to see the larger picture about how we bring the boards [interdisciplinary councils] together to look at our practice."

Restructured Management of Nursing Services

Changes in the management and organizational structure of nursing services have begun to occur as a result of the work of the CNO and others as they restructure the broader patient care delivery system. The organizational design of clinical divisions and patient care units is being challenged and reconsidered. New designs, called communities of care, have been introduced and have led to a reconsideration of the overall managerial and organizational structure. Some nurse managers interviewed considered the change in structure simply to be a substitute of one form of organizational structure for another, without any real change in the way the organization will work.

Specifically, the nurse manager and nursing director roles are being altered. Not all nurse managers or nursing directors report to the CNO, a point that was of concern to the CNO as well as to the nurse leaders and managers. The long-term effect of this change is what concerns the CNO. She indicated that it might be workable because of the people in place now, but if she or any of the other vice presidents were to leave, she asked rhetorically: "What will that mean for the future of nursing?" A nurse manager indicated that this change in reporting relationships means that the professional dimension of the structure needs to be even stronger.

The nursing director role, previously titled nurse leader and consultant, has been eliminated in some areas and in other areas vastly expanded in responsibilities. Paralleling in some ways the changes in the CNO role, the nursing director now assumes broader responsibility for program management, finances, and patient care service integration. The title given to this expanded role has changed to director, patient care services. As their workload increases, the nursing directors' focus is no longer solely on nursing, and their presence to nurse managers and clinical nursing staff is, like the CNO's, much less than in the past.

All these changes have led nurse managers to feel that their role is being challenged faster than most others. A focus on practice development for the nursing staff and day-to-day operations of the unit remain expectations of the nurse manager role, but there also is a shift from unit-specific responsibility to a broader scope of practice and organizational work as they assume greater responsibility for more units. Nurse managers feel the pressure of this change, especially as they become more involved in the organization's finances and not just the budgets of their own units. More is being decentralized to the nurse manager level, including more interface with other disciplines and, in some circumstances, across the system. Until recently, these functions were considered the responsibility of the nursing director or even the CNO.

One positive result of this change in the functioning of the nurse manager was expressed by the medical director, who indicated that the respect and recognition for nursing has grown as a result of the increased strength of the nurse manager role. Yet, nurse managers expressed concern about the direct impact of organizational changes on their ability to function well in their role. The CNO's increased distance from the daily work of the nurse managers is of concern, although they appear to understand its necessity in developing the CNO role's influence in broader organizational issues. It is, however, the perceived loss of the needed administrative and clinical support previously provided as part of the director of nursing position that compounds their concern.

The CEO indicated that the expansion of nursing director responsibility, with a simultaneous reduction in the number of directors, relates to the desire to become more efficient. This, he stated, will be achieved by increasing nurse manager authority and responsibility.[2] He further indicated that it is the clinical background of nursing as well as the willingness of nurses to learn the management side of operations that leads to this organizational decision.

With the decline in the number of nursing director positions in the organizational structure, the nurse managers' scope of responsibility has expanded, removing them further and for longer periods of time from the needs of the clinical nursing staff. The expectations for nurse managers to be involved in broader activities of the organization have increased, and they feel that they need help to accomplish these as well as the previous expectations. A former nurse manager expressed the tension of this role change as follows:

> NURSE MANAGER: So that's one of the biggest tensions I feel . . . and I'm not sure if I'm a proponent for that layer [that is, director] being gone because as a manager, one of the things I struggled with constantly and one of the main reasons I'm not a manager any longer is that I could not do what I felt needed to be done in terms of the individual day-to-day mentoring work with the staff. It's a 24-hour-a-day business, 7 days a week. To touch and to interact and to be present for that many staff is overwhelming.
> INTERVIEWER: How many would it be?
> NURSE MANAGER: For me, and I had one partner, I partnered with one other person, and we had about 230 staff. That's incredible to think about, the total operation including the financial pieces and all that was overwhelming. And one of the biggest benefits that I always felt that I had from the nurse leader consultant [director] was that was a person that I could consult with, who could help me by removing some barriers that I had identified but was having a difficult time with.

There also is a feeling that change has brought chaos. A number of organizational designs have been proposed and are in various stages of implementation, with transition in roles happening at the same time. All this tends to increase the level of ambiguity and, thus, tension in the organization. Nurse managers expressed feelings of conflict. The concern they voiced is for the quality of care and the professional development of staff. The latter has become increasingly important as the competencies needed in the changed environment of patient care have changed.

The change in knowledge and skills needed to do the job successfully was addressed by one nurse manager in referencing her own work and the job realities she now faces. Feeling an immense sense of accountability and challenge, she is no longer as sure of herself as she once was, even though she is very seasoned in her role and well prepared by both education and experience:

> Well, you know, there obviously have been a lot of changes, and there are far less of us than there used to be, and I think the requirements of the people in these roles range from somebody who needs to have some level of clinical proficiency to understand the business, to being

pretty greatly versed in group process, change process and innovation and quality, and you name it. We are basically where the buck stops on a 24-hour basis. It's been a very challenging thing even for somebody such as myself. I have a master's degree in a clinical specialty and felt like I had a good background to do the role, but, boy, you find out quickly because the world changes.

As the nurse manager's workload changes, the need for a CNO to design a system that will provide administrative support and counsel increases. One nurse manager described this need as follows:

I've seen my role change. I've seen a number of us diminish, and the workload has only become more complex, so when I think about what I need from a vice president, I still think I have a need for a connection with a director-level position. . . . My boss functions in a consultative capacity, not superinvolved in the operations. It's more of an oversight, consultative role and I find that is very valuable. I know when I need her for the major urgencies, for the things that come up, the ethical dilemmas where I need another mind to help me determine if I am on the right track or maybe I am not on the right track, and I find that invaluable. So as our organization has started to change, that is one of the roles that is changed. . . . It's really much more of an advisory, consultative capacity that I need. I just need a mind that I know *gets* the big picture and who understands the business and says, "Yeah, I think you're right" or "I think this is a good way to approach an extremely complex and difficult issue." The things we are dealing with have become more and more complex in terms of ethics, complexity, politics, policy.

Clinical Staff-Administrative Relationships

Throughout the interviews with nurse managers and nurse leaders during the on-site visit to White Hospital, reference was made to the high relationship needs of the clinical nursing staff. One manager expressed it this way: "Even if they [nurses] don't talk to you, they want to see you or feel that they can." The significant impact that nurse managers have on allocating resources, identifying practice dimensions, helping identify high-risk situations in the care process, and developing processes for quality management were all noted as part of the important role relationships that managers and clinical staff share.

Added to the above is the need staff have, as nurturers themselves, for nurturing—a responsibility many of the nurse managers interviewed felt they were no longer fulfilling because of the expansion of their work responsibilities. This greatly concerns nurse managers, and it was not uncommon for descriptions of this change in staff relationships to be conveyed intensely and emotionally. When speaking of changed relationships, one nurse manager said she has "felt more like a target and less like a leader." Although she believes she has learned a lot through her changing role and has gained more respect for other departments, this has occurred at the expense of her relationships with her own nursing staff: "It's the hardest thing I've ever done in my whole life from an emotional standpoint. The work itself is not hard, but the emotional toll it takes has been great."

Another nurse manager described one serious impact of her role change as being removed from the unit and the staff who need her presence. Staff are capable, but they have high expectations that they will have consultation when needed and a nurse manager who can monitor staff development needs and quality of care. These expectations were considered appropriate, especially in light of the following observation of still another nurse manager, who suggested that substantial changes have affected the clinical nursing staff as well. Their workload now precludes them from having time to look up critical information needed for the complexity of care needs they now encounter. They have less access to the nurse manager, a significant resource loss to the clinical nursing staff at a time they need it most. Role conflict was evident in her description—not guilt but, rather, a feeling of hopelessness regarding her availability to staff.

Within this context, the CNO role is viewed as an essential way for the nurse manager and the clinical nursing staff to connect with the larger organization. The need is to help establish for them that the work they are doing is consistent with larger organizational needs and direction, as well as with overall nursing practice standards. The need to maintain practice standards seemed to be increasingly important to those nurse managers who have taken on responsibility for managing other professionals. Many nurse managers now have, and feel accountable for, multiple relationships and interactions that go beyond the nursing department, even if the reporting line is drawn only to that department. The desire to ensure that those professionals, as well as nurse professionals, have the opportunity to set their own standards of practice and retain professional identity also was expressed by nurse managers during the interview process. This corroborates the important role often ascribed to the CNO for visibility, comfort, and presence through personal interaction and communication.

Relationship of the CNO Role to High-Quality Patient Care

Although it was not within the scope of this study to examine the results of role change on patient care, the concern about quality and safety in care was referred to frequently during the interviews at White Hospital. This organization considers the CNO role to be an important variable in achieving its mission of providing high-quality patient care and services. The CEO indicated that nurses are the communicators and evaluators of patient care and that the reason the vice president for patient services is a nurse, rather than a member of another clinical discipline, is because of the known dedication of nurses to the care of the patient and nursing's constancy with the patient. The medical director supported this view as he discussed the important role of the CNO in patient advocacy and determining clinical excellence in the organization. From the perspective of this physician, nurses were "literally responsible for the quality of patient care."

Although members of the nursing leadership and management groups suggest there is an increasing need for patient advocacy in the current health care environment, they also are concerned that the CNO's expanding responsibilities will dilute her ability to remain focused on that need. As one put it:

> The value of nursing, as you know, is that we are the ones that are advocates for the patients' response. . . . It's not just the compartmentalization of disease or the drugs or the physical therapy, but we have that [overall] perspective that is concerned with the whole issue. And I am deeply concerned. It's not the discipline thing that I need to hold on to, but it's the idea of someone being an advocate for the whole of patient care and I don't know that any one office has that. And we have struggled here because we have seen shakiness as the reorganization occurred that it could happen that the vice president for patient care became another operations line, like every other operations line.

The previous CNO of White Hospital articulated the importance of developing good, complementary interdisciplinary relationships in the care of patients. The outcomes of patient care depend on this, she says, because it provides a holistic approach to care and helps reduce the margin of error by setting up different checks and balances. A nurse manager concurred with this notion by saying that integration is the goal—integration for patients in planning and giving care. This is the way she believes the system will be able to provide patients what they need in an efficient manner.

In the end, it seems that although the concerns of nursing management and leadership staff over the changes occurring in their roles and that of the CNO are substantial, staff are most interested in preserving high-quality patient care. Interdisciplinary care delivery is viewed as a positive goal to work toward in this environment in order to maintain the quality of care. Their belief that the CNO role is important in this process is summed up by one nurse manager as follows:

I think there would probably be a riot [if there were no chief nurse role]. I believe staff see the importance, as I do, that nursing is a huge component of patient care and affects most significantly the patient experience and that there needs to be a person—articulate, smart—to be representing that as decisions are made at high levels. And I think there would be a lot of concern about who'd be watching out for the patient, as well as what is going on with the practice, if there isn't that person there. I think it's actually more important now than it's ever been to make sure that the interests of the patients are being serviced.

CONCLUDING REMARKS

Access to White Hospital was granted with graciousness and openness beginning with the initial contact with the CEO of the White Consolidated Health System, who immediately provided the names of the hospital's CEO and CNO and information about changes that had occurred in the CNO position. The current CNO and CEO of the hospital did the same. As the nature of the study was discussed, the CEO even suggested interviewing the former CNO, who now held a position at the corporate level. The CNO was equally gracious and quite excited when asked to expand the interviewing process to include nurse managers. Throughout the two days of the site visit, everyone involved demonstrated a deep sense of commitment and professionalism.

What the interview data obtained at White Hospital revealed most clearly was how very important it is to have an understanding of the history of the organization over time. The changes taking place at White Hospital sound much like those taking place in many other hospitals in the country today, but knowing the organization's history provides a different level of insight when assessing the efficacy of these changes.

This story of change brought to light how sensitive transitions in leadership are—and how closely members of the organization watch or examine the actions and behaviors of leaders, especially new leaders. The CNO's integrator role is clearly dominant in this hospital, and yet because of personal style, it is not as easily recognized by some members of the nursing staff. They need time to trust that this CNO shares their values.

Notes

1. The hospital CEO suggested interviewing the previous CNO, who had been in the position for slightly more than five years before moving to the corporate level of the organization to work across the system on

quality improvement issues. The incumbent CNO made the same suggestion and developed the interview schedule to ensure the past CNO's availability. Without the past CNO's inclusion in the study, the story of White Hospital's change process would have been somewhat incomplete.

2. A proposed organizational chart indicates the potential change of the clinical nurse manager title to that of patient care manager. Although not proposed as such, concern was expressed that disciplines other than nursing could hold that position, exacerbating concerns voiced by the nurse managers about the effects of the current managerial role changes on clinical nursing staff.

6

Blue Hospital Case Study

INTRODUCTION

Founded in 1915, Blue Hospital is a 600-bed tertiary, acute care hospital located in a metropolitan area it has served for most of this century. The current administration is very proud of the hospital's academic and research mission, which provides postgraduate education for about 650 medical residents and fellows. In 1996 Blue Hospital closed its diploma school of nursing and began a university nursing program affiliation.

Demographics and Features

Blue Hospital is one of seven hospitals in an IDS that spans a large geographic area and is divided into six regional delivery systems, each of which has a medical director and an administrator. The system is 40 percent managed care, which is expected to increase in the near future.

In addition to the hospital component, the IDS is composed of multiple other facilities, including 45 suburban satellite ambulatory care centers, two HMOs (one having about 450,000 members), and extensive emergency care services that expand far beyond the annual 92,000 emergency unit visits experienced by Blue Hospital. The system also includes a large, influential multispecialty medical group practice and systemwide employs nearly 20,000 people. There are 900 salaried MDs.

At the time of the study, it was rumored that a merger or affiliation might take place between Blue Hospital and other area hospitals once considered competitors. Building such relationships was considered to be necessary in light of the growing possibility that the for-profit health care management industry was about to emerge in the area. Thus, there was a sense of pending change within the immediate environment that would have an impact on Blue Hospital.

Environmental Context

With a 21.6 percent HMO penetration, the metropolitan area in which Blue Hospital resides is not in the top 26 large markets that have 25 percent or greater HMO penetration (Interstudy Competitive Edge 1996). The area is dominated by a single industry whose unionized employees historically have resisted involvement in managed care health plans. However, since 1994 the industry's health care benefit costs have declined as a result of its success in encouraging some of its employees to enroll in the less costly HMO and PPO plans (Singer 1996).

Also of interest is that even though the area's health care market has been strongly influenced by the negotiations of this single industry and its union employees, the business sector overall has not applied the level of activity and pressure to the market that has occurred in other areas of the country (Ginsburg 1996).

Hospital capacity has not been reduced by much in this area, nor has there been much consolidation. The metropolitan service area comprises 58 hospitals, 7 IDSs, 8 HMOs, and 12 PPOs (Singer 1996). In an effort to further reduce the cost of health care benefits, the area's major industry is focusing on wellness programs and working closely with area hospitals and physicians to achieve better care outcomes for beneficiaries (Singer 1996).

Restructuring

Many of those interviewed for this study indicated that the restructuring of Blue Hospital's care delivery system and clinical operations, although anticipated, had not yet fully occurred. They and others provided an overview of a pilot program that has been used to demonstrate the envisioned changes as well as some insights on preparatory change that has begun. The planned changes focus on two efforts: patient-focused care and product line restructuring.

Patient-Focused Care   A plan for redesigning the care delivery model has been developed and implemented within a pilot unit of the hospital to test the design's applicability for the larger organization. The major component of this redesigned care delivery model includes decentralizing as many services as possible to the patient care unit. Some facility reconstruction has taken place to accommodate the design, but the major redesign is in changing many of the ancillary or support roles in patient care. For example, six roles, each of which had formally worked out of a central department, were merged into one and deployed to the patient care unit. This process, called *multiskilling*, required hospital-wide education and training in preparation for the model's widespread application. Multiskilling also requires that nurse managers assume responsibility for a broader group of professional and nonprofessional staff who will provide their services locally under the direction of an RN or within the geographic area of the nurse manager's responsibility.

In addition, some nurse mangers have had their scope of responsibility expanded to include more than a single patient care unit. This has occurred in the clinical nurse specialist role as well. For both these roles, expansion across units is expected to continue, although the nurse manager's responsibility is expected to remain within the same product line.

Product Line Restructuring   Product line restructuring is the plan for Blue Hospital. This is in line with an overall system plan for applying the model of product line management to the six regions of the IDS. In other words, regional boundaries exist within which, but not generally beyond which, the product lines can be marketed. According to the hospital CEO, this is a strategy established with the intent of avoiding competition within the IDS itself. Product lines, however, are expected to cross the boundaries of the hospital and other parts of the system, focusing on the continuum of services as well as the acute episode that requires hospital services.

Blue Hospital's product line restructuring took place after the interviews for this study were conducted. It reorganized the traditional administrative structure of departments by eliminating most central departmental functions, including those of nursing. In the process, four vice presidents were identified as vice presidents of patient care services. Now, a product line manager who has complete authority for the entire product (for example, women's health) reports to one of the assigned vice presidents for patient care services. Two of the four vice presidents are nurses, one of whom is the former vice president for nursing. She also continues to hold the official responsibility as CNO. Without a central department of nursing, the CNO role serves as both figurehead and spokesperson for nurses and manages the remaining central professional nursing functions that relate to staff development and research activities. The CNO also chairs the coordinating council of the nursing shared governance committee structure, which was carried over from the traditional departmental structure as one way to coordinate nursing standards hospitalwide.

CHANGE AT BLUE HOSPITAL

"Anticipatory change" is the best way to describe Blue Hospital's environment at the time of the site visit in June 1996. Much of the change that had taken place up to that point seemed to be in preparation for a larger, more substantial organizational restructuring expected to occur later in the year. Planning for a product line approach to clinical services and developing models for patient-focused care were the primary components of this anticipated change.

Simultaneously, the image of nursing was improving at Blue Hospital as nurses made changes to enhance their professional role within the organization. Nursing as a discipline had not been viewed as a powerful influence within this organization, although many cited the need for this to be so. In part, the reason for this was that until recently the nursing department had lacked the resources to function with little more than a task-oriented focus toward patient care. Because the RN ratio was low (approximately 30 percent), additional resources were made to the department's staffing budget. Increasing staffing resources of varying skill mix sets the stage for the discussion of change at Blue Hospital. This event has had implications for the nursing staff's perception of the CNO role in terms of her relationship with hospital administration and the nurses' ability to provide patient care.

Nine years ago, the incumbent CNO came to Blue Hospital to take on the challenge of developing a strong nursing department. At the time, the department had a very high RN turnover rate (more than 30 percent). Moreover, there was a very high ratio of LPNs (about a third of the staff), and about 40 percent of the staff were nonlicensed personnel. This situation existed in an era when many other hospitals had primarily all-RN staffs. The last class of the diploma school of nursing had graduated only a few weeks before the site visit. This fact influenced the educational preparation of the RN workforce available to Blue Hospital. Since then, the hospital has begun a formal affiliation with a local university school of nursing and the dean of that school will interface at the system level of the organization.

Influence of Patient-Focused Care and Total Quality Management

The current change activities began, in part, with the CNO's development of a proposal for the planning grant Strengthening Hospital Nursing: A Project to Improve Patient Care, funded by the RWJ and Pew Charitable Trust Foundations. She received a one-year planning grant but was not as successful in obtaining one of the 20 five-year grants subsequently provided. Nevertheless, the grant provided the impetus to do some rethinking about the way the hospital designed its delivery of care. When a new CEO arrived in 1991, the CNO used the opportunity to introduce him to the concepts of patient-focused care, the elements that had come from the work of the planning grant. He took this seriously, attended a national conference on patient-focused care, and became committed to the potential this design held for the organization. He now is leading the change process by chairing a steering committee on patient-focused care. In addition, a number of planning and redesign groups are in place, all of which are attempting to accomplish redesign efforts at the patient care unit level of the organization.

During the interview, the CEO agreed with the CNO's assessment that there had been no infrastructure for nursing in 1991. There was no teamwork, the collaborative management of care and services did not exist, and no one, including nurses, seemed to understand the professional role of the RN. When he became CEO, the CNO's previous documentation of nurse staffing issues led him to conclude that a benchmarking consultant would be helpful. Thus, a benchmarking study was carried out by a major national firm, the results of which supported the fact that the hospital's nurse staffing was significantly different from that of other similar organizations. The CNO developed a proposal that successfully added about $3 million for staffing to the nursing budget. The CEO credited this as being the change needed to move forward with collaboration and the promotion of the RN role in the management of care delivery.

Further, the CEO indicated that one of the major reasons for the change in thinking at Blue Hospital was his own involvement in the program of patient-focused care. He was taken with the customer satisfaction focus of this care delivery design. He said that the design really represented a total quality improvement (TQM) program that could involve the whole hospital, and the potential efficiencies of this process excited him. No doubt, this underscores the value of having leadership from the top of the organization actively involved in order to ensure that change will take place on a broad scale.

According to the nurse managers interviewed, TQM was perceived to be an important catalyst for change. The process, which began about four years before, was cited by the nurse managers as not only making things change in the hospital but also providing the opportunity for greater interaction with others. TQM focuses on what the patient wants and needs, and forces people to look across departments and disciplines, thereby enhancing the teamwork experience.

Change in CNO Responsibilities

The CNO described her scope of responsibility in terms of areas managed in her department or services reporting to her, such as pastoral services and inpatient units. She was clear that her appointment as CNO had been for inpatient nursing only and that even today there is no central leadership for the ambulatory nursing component at Blue Hospital. Below, she offers her perception of the reasons why nursing was split up and defined as the number of units or services managed:

Nursing is, well, you measure your power by the size of budget, by the size of FTEs, and the amount of information you have. So who-ever controls nursing controls a major portion of the workforce. I mean nursing is the infantry of health care, and you can't take the hill without her. So it's much better if I [as an administrator] have the ER, then my piece of the pie is bigger and my amount of money is bigger, and so it really is directly related. And hospitals and health care are mostly a male-dominated culture, and males are not like females. We are more egalitarian, and we attack our own when someone tries to get out of that egalitarian equalness. When some-one is less equal and tries to be higher, then we go after them. But males, they don't expect egalitarianism, they expect hierarchy; and even if you are a VP and you are all the same VPs, they know from football that there is the first-string quarterback, the second-string quarterback, the third-string quarterback, and the bench sitter. And, so even though you are all VPs, they, in their minds, have a hierar-chy, and they are always jockeying for hierarchy of dominance and where they are in that hierarchy. This is overgeneralization, but it comes from long, hard experience.

Organizational power and gender-related management style are recurring themes in the interview with the CNO. They are the reasons she gave for the way nursing was distributed among hospital adminis-trators, including herself, and the way her overall responsibility was defined. She suggested that gender issues influence several other aspects of organizational work relationships as well. Although the issues related to gender differences have been described often with regard to nurses and physicians (that is, a predominately female pro-fession operating vis-à-vis a predominately male profession), the dis-cussion with this CNO raises the question of the extent or relevance of gender-related issues in the administration of health care services.

Blue Hospital's CEO also described the organizational structure of nursing and the CNO's responsibilities as inpatient only, characterizing ambulatory nursing as having been "spun off." He spoke of the JCAHO and other regulatory agencies' requirement for a CNO "figurehead" to ensure that quality is consistent throughout the organization. In light of that, he said, and because the systemwide CEO places a high value on nursing, the incumbent CNO sits on the senior operating team at the corporate level. The question this discussion raises is, How can the CNO implement consistency in patient care quality and nursing practice if she has no formalized organizational relationship with those in practice at the local level? The system-level operating team spoken of by the CEO deals with broad policy issues, not with the specifics of operational management. The opportunity to design, facilitate, or implement nursing practice systems is absent in the ambulatory setting, and thus the impact of the CNO role is limited.

Because of this, the CNO indicated she has tried to work through the back doors to improve ambulatory care. She does this because she lacks authority within the system to work directly with ambulatory nurses. One of the consequences of having a CNO role that is limited in scope is the potential for inconsistent standards for patient care and services across the system.

When discussing the organizational boundaries of having only inpatient units as the defining elements of the CNO's responsibilities, a senior corporate officer suggested that the lack of a strong nursing leadership presence could be related to the traditionally strong leadership role played by physicians in this organization from its beginning. Historically, there were never "downtown practices." The physicians were always present in the hospital, and for the first 60 years of the hospital's history, nursing and medicine probably had a good partnership. It was when the hospital became something else, part of what now is understood to be an IDS, with greater presence in ambulatory care in the suburbs, that nursing lost its leadership edge.

It seems that when the executive leadership of the IDS worked to develop a systems approach, their strength and focus went to the system and the flagship hospital was, in essence, left without CEO leadership. Nor did other leadership step forward from nursing, medicine, or administration, which resulted in a period of "floundering." All this, it was said, took away from the cohesive and synergistic nursing program and physician partnership of the past. Nurses became the hospital's inpatient care providers and specialty care sitters.

Considering the current trend in health care away from use of acute inpatient care settings to increased use of ambulatory and community services, the absence of nursing leadership for patient care in the latter settings is likely to become more significant in the future. Thus, a new paradigm that incorporates nurses as care providers might need to be developed for ambulatory care; otherwise, nurses will simply be moving into existing physician ambulatory practices a technical support role as the model for nursing practice.

LEADERSHIP DIMENSIONS AND THE CNO ROLE

The analysis of interview data obtained at Blue Hospital looked for evidence of the three areas of organizational and professional leadership identified as forming the conceptual foundation for CNO role expectations as integrator, communicator, and designer.

CNO as Integrator

Some of the evidence sought concerned the CNO's influence with other groups or role partners—that is, her influence in the organization as a liaison leader. The CNO described her peers as the CFO and four other vice presidents. As a team, the six of them regularly meet with the hospital CEO and periodically go on retreats. Although her relationship with this group is still developing under the current CEO's leadership, it is a far cry from the dysfunctional team relationship she had experienced previously. In fact, for the first few years of her tenure, her relationship with the previous CEO was strained and difficult to the extent that she felt impeded in her attempts to make the needed changes that she and the current CEO have begun to implement subsequently. Moreover, her difficulties with the previous CEO adversely affected her working relationships with other members of senior management. Because the current CEO places greater value on her work, she receives more recognition within the senior management team as a whole. This situation indicates the critical nature of organizational recognition, both functionally and structurally. Titles and placement within the organization are of limited use if the relationships developed fail to recognize or value the work.

The nurse managers interviewed identified the CNO leadership role as important in ensuring nursing's involvement in the larger strategic planning activities of the organization. The CNO's leadership was cited as essential in helping the organization achieve its goals, and the CNO-CEO partnership was viewed as necessary to get things done for patient care.

The CNO also indicated that she understood the importance of integration to the organization. Although she readily admitted being less visible to staff and somewhat tired of working long days, she said that she relies on the organizational design of a strong nursing management team to help with both visibility and integration. She works closely with nurse managers and associate directors, and it is through them that she expects integration will take place.

Although both the CNO and the CEO described the various committees and meetings the CNO attends, the extent of her influence as a strong integrator in this organization was unclear. There was no palpable evidence of liaison leadership during the site visit and the interviews, and the impression was that perhaps the integrator role was carried out through her work with the associate directors.

CNO as Communicator

When the CNO stepped into her role several years ago, she felt it essential to establish a visible identity with staff so as to gain their trust and establish her credibility. She made herself available at various times, meeting with staff on the off-shifts as well as the day shift. However, during the current period of change, the CNO, as well as other members of the nursing management staff, acknowledged a decline in her visibility and communication with staff, and both she and the staff expressed their concern about it. It is an odd twist in that a period of uncertainty would seem to be the time that CNO visibility would be most needed.

Some years previously, the CNO designed a system of shared governance specifically to address nursing practice development. Practice councils and committees for all units continue to serve as a vehicle for communication between the clinical nursing staff and the hospital's management and nursing administration. The CNO suggested that this system of shared governance would be the way a central standard-setting process would continue when the nursing department is removed and a product line organizational structure is implemented. However, at the time of this study, no plans were in place showing how these multiple governance councils would interface with the hospital's senior management, nor was it clear that a central chief nursing officer role would continue. A postinterview phone conversation with the CNO revealed that the product line organizational structure has been implemented and that she has assumed responsibility as vice president for two of the product lines and has retained the CNO designation for the organization. The CNO designation does not include operational responsibility for nursing practice across the organization but, rather, serves to identify the individual who will represent nursing in various forums. The CNO retains responsibility for nursing staff development, research, and quality but has only limited access to the staff in a central way in the organization. Chairing the coordinating council of the shared governance model is the established vehicle for her to do this, although the council members comprise only a small number of representative staff. It seems probable that in a product line organizational structure established without either a central nursing department or a CNO with central authority for nursing practice across the system, the CNO's visibility and information-sharing role will be, at best, circumscribed.

CNO as Designer

The important role of architect of the institution was discussed by the hospital's corporate-level senior vice president, who indicated that it is the CNO position, more than any other, that has that responsibility. He stated that this is so because the design of patient care delivery systems and the clinical teams involved in care delivery have a special nature about them and the CNO is "the best person positioned to really produce the delivery model that is going to sustain us."

Sustaining the organization to meet its mission of high-quality patient care is a responsibility that CNOs assume in hospital organizations. They carry out these expectations in various ways. For example, when the CNO at Blue Hospital was unable to generate support from the previous CEO for increased staffing, she tried another strategy: She designed and received funding for a computerized nursing informatics system that was tied to the organization's financial system. This system reduced much of the RNs' paperwork and helped to galvanize staff around the standards of care and nursing practice that were needed. This made the change process visible and made the staff feel more involved with the change. The CNO also managed to redesign some of the FTEs in the nursing budget, using them to employ clinical nurse specialists (advanced practice nurses) whom she moved to patient care units to help shape the nurse manager role. This outcome was achieved, and the nurse manager role now assumes far greater responsibility for all aspects of the unit's functioning, both clinical and business. Designing the system to use advanced practice nurses as agents of change was a successful strategy that might prove useful again in the current development of a new care delivery model.

In the interview process, nurse managers voiced their concern about the potential changes that might result from Blue Hospital's current redesign planning. They believed that however the system was designed, one person still would need to have an overall vision of where the nursing department should be heading. They felt that this person should be a nurse executive, for it was the understanding of the current CNO that brought respect and stature to other nursing management roles, such as their own, and consequently allowed them to be more effective in the organization.

SYSTEM LEADERSHIP AND THE CNO ROLE

In one interview, the absence of nursing leadership was cited by a senior system leader as making a difference to both the organization and the system. He believes there needs to be a focal point for nursing leadership in the organization. At the same time, however, he wondered what really needed to be centrally guided by a CNO as the professional "silos" break down and the organization becomes more centered around diseases and processes.

Ambivalence about how to incorporate this central leadership role for nursing at the hospital level is what came through in this interview. However, the senior corporate leader was clear in his belief that there is a need at the system's corporate level for more nursing representation. A Chief Nurse Executive Council, consisting of the CNOs of each of the system's hospitals, meets and is chaired by the CNO of the flagship hospital. However, the various clinical business units remained underrepresented in nursing leadership when it comes time for strategic planning retreats.

The CNO indicated that she is involved at least twice a month with the system-level CEO and senior vice president for hospital integration. She attends the corporate retreats and sits on the corporate quality committee, although she is not the only CNO within the system who attends.

The perceived void of nursing leadership at the corporate level is now being addressed with the addition, at some of the management forums, of the dean of the school of nursing, who has recently become affiliated with the overall system. It is intended that she, along with the CNO of the flagship hospital, will have linkages not just with the acute side of the system, but also with the ambulatory side and the care delivery models that are evolving in both settings. This conversation suggested that the corporate organization wants to elevate and increase nursing leadership within the system, but to do so through use of nursing education at the system level rather than by designing a stronger leadership role at the hospital level.

Impact on the Organization of the CNO Role Change

At the time of the study visit to Blue Hospital, the CNO's title was still vice president for nursing, although a change in title was anticipated with the future introduction of a product line structure. As noted previously, a follow-up phone conversation with the CNO confirmed that her title and responsibilities had in fact changed since the interview. However, at the time of the site visit, product line restructuring was still in the preimplementation stage and only a few steps had been taken to set patient-focused care in motion. Thus, the organizational impact discussed below describes the hospital and the CNO role prior to the change to product line organization and the changes in the CNO role and title.

The change process at Blue Hospital placed an emphasis on breaking down the silos of the organization. The nursing department was considered a silo and not expected to remain as a department following implementation of a product line structure, nor was it expected that there would be a combined patient care service department.

When discussing the organization's anticipated change to a product line structure, the CNO of Blue Hospital expressed conflict, believing on the one hand that the traditional nursing department is outdated and represents a silo approach to patient care delivery and on the other hand that there needs "to be a keeper of the keys for quality in nursing," which underscores the importance of a central role for nursing. She even vacillated about the need for the CNO position itself.

The CEO also discussed his view of the nursing department of the future, indicating the need to integrate services. He indicated that a CNO is still needed to relate to the clinical staff for monitoring the credentialing and reappointment processes for nursing staff and for setting standards and clinical expectations. He suggested that these functions need to be designed in a decentralized manner for the future and sees the changes occurring in steps. A "nursing champion" would remain— someone who would keep the quality of nursing high, ensure standards across the product lines, and seek the same quality of care throughout the organization. This CEO recognized the potential for fragmentation with product lines if they were not centrally connected in some fashion. He also wanted product lines to be integrated across the system, not just within the inpatient areas of the acute care hospital, suggesting that the organization must form concentric circles that integrate collaboratively for the product lines so as to ensure consistency in the standard of care provided. How to do this, however, was not yet developed, although he had some thoughts about the kind of person needed: "So, ultimately, I see that as kind of a growing need, and obviously the type of person required for that is going to have to have more than just your basic management skills. [It will need to be] someone who has the leadership ability, who can influence and rally people together, who really spans a whole integrated system and creates some infrastructure to carry these things out."

Moreover, this individual's organizational placement was not clear in the CEO's mind. He predicted that some of the change would be incremental and that, initially, the current CNO would be charged with creating this model at the same time that she served as senior administrator for one or more product lines.

The impression gleaned from the interviews with the CEO and the corporate vice president mentioned earlier is that, ultimately, nursing would be integrated across all product lines as though it were a product line itself, with the overall vision and direction coming from a new nursing leadership role yet to be established at the corporate level of the IDS. Whether this role would be carried out by one person or many was yet to be determined. The CEO suggested that the sheer size of the RN workforce for the system might require multiple leadership roles at the system level.

Associate directors of nursing spoke about the need for breaking down departmental silos and understanding the business of the whole organization. They indicated that, to date, the main change in their own role has been to attend more interdisciplinary meetings and to develop a broader view of the larger organization. They had no idea what their role might be in a product line structure. The roles that had begun to change, they felt, were those of the nurse manager and the clinical nurse specialist. Expansion of the workload for these roles had begun, with some nurse managers and clinical specialists assuming responsibility for more than one unit.

The associate directors also talked about their responsibility for developing the nursing staff, helping them learn how to make the change, and providing them with guidance and support. To a large extent, the change they seemed to refer to in this discussion seemed less directed at the organizational restructuring of product line than at the early development of a professional model of nursing practice with decentralized decision making, competency building, and practice development.

When discussing the organizational changes expected with product line and patient-focused care delivery, the associate directors of nursing believed that this structure could be carried out in the short term without destroying the philosophy that they and others in the organization hold of putting the "patient first," as long as the current nonnursing senior leadership is in place. In particular, they felt there would be a risk for the future if the leadership of the current CEO were lost.

Management and Administration of Nursing Services

The system vice president interviewed indicated that all line management positions at Blue Hospital were being either stretched in terms of scope of responsibility or eliminated organizationally. Examining changes in the nurse manager role there was complicated by the fact that the nurse managers had only recently been given responsibilities that other hospitals have long considered part of their role. Increasing the numbers of RN staff began this change by placing a greater emphasis on delivery site leadership and decision making. To date, the change felt by the nurse managers relates more to this than to patient-focused care or product line restructuring.

During their interviews, members of the nurse manager group indicated that they expected even more changes in their role under patient-focused care because they would have responsibility for managing members of other departments. This would increase both the number of FTEs to supervise and their individual administrative responsibilities. Some already had experienced a change as a result of the early implementation of patient-focused care on their units, with increased responsibility for evaluating various kinds of staff and their performance. Quality control responsibilities, they indicated, extended to tasks redeployed from other departments. For example, they would be expected to know what a quality electrocardiogram is, as well as how to evaluate housekeeping's performance in cleaning a bed or bathroom following discharge. Previously, these responsibilities had belonged to the central departments.

Discussions with both the nurse managers and the associate directors again suggested conflict about the new responsibilities. On the one hand, they recognized the advantage to learning more about the work of others, including getting to know the whole system and knowing whom to call on to get things done; on the other hand, however, they were ambivalent about the new responsibilities because the time involved in managing additional areas would take time away from helping the nursing staff to improve and develop their clinical practice, a first step toward ensuring quality in patient care.

A major change for nurse managers is their involvement as representatives of nursing in a variety of meetings or other forums both on and off campus. Some nurse managers have greater systemwide responsibility than others, mostly related to their clinical specialty knowledge. In many ways, their systemwide representation is greater than the CNO's because of its specialized clinical planning focus. However, nurse managers expressed some frustration about this new representative role. They feel isolated as they assume increasing levels of independent management responsibility, yet also feel they *must* attend meetings to ensure that the voice of nursing is heard. As product lines are developed as more independent business units and a central nursing department are no longer in place, this sense of isolation will increase. How the nurse managers are being mentored and developed for these new responsibilities could not be answered by those interviewed.

According to the nurse managers, the changes have brought more formality to the organization. For example, it once was easy to meet with whomever they needed to, including the CNO. But now, with everyone's role expanding, they have to make an appointment—and still risk being bumped. This is as true with other nurse managers as it is across the organization. Everyone's schedule has been stretched to include more meetings, yet the quality of their interactions has diminished. Examination of one nurse manager's appointment calendar showed that at the beginning of the year, she had about eight meetings scheduled during the entire month. Her schedule now is up to seven meetings a day, without a repeat of anything in the month. Others agreed that the number of meetings has increased dramatically. As a result, time management has become a problem, and the nurse managers are worried about what will happen as they continue to spend more time off the unit and away from the clinical nursing staff.

Clinical Staff–Administrative Relationship

The nurse manager's span of control is expanding not only because of increasing responsibilities of representation at the system level, but also because the number of nurse managers is decreasing. As nurse managers leave, they are not being replaced and the trend is for the remaining nurse managers to take on responsibility for more than one unit. Thus, nurse managers are moving further away from the work of the clinical nursing staff, despite the continued need for someone to oversee clinical management of the units and to help staff continue to develop their expertise in patient care. The clinical manager's work includes coordination, collaboration with other disciplines, development of methods to evaluate outcomes, and the all-important daily problem solving. All this requires an individual who understands the nature of clinical care and how the processes work.

The nurse managers at Blue Hospital emphasized the fact that clinical nursing staff need to know that someone in authority understands what they are doing and hears their concerns about patient care. This discussion highlighted the intensity and complexity of patient care. Patient care involves not only the correct performance of tasks and procedures, but also confirmation, support, and dialogue with others about what is happening in the process of caregiving and the patient response to it. Clinicians working in potentially life-threatening situations with patients and families need to have their judgment validated.

The nurse manager role expansion really comes to light in clinical staff performance evaluations, according to the nurse managers interviewed. Nurse managers no longer feel able to do as much for or with the nursing staff because their work has become much more administrative; they are more involved with paperwork and less involved with the clinical unit's daily operations. Thus, evaluating how the nursing staff are performing in this environment is increasingly difficult. Many expressed the hope that the assistant nurse manager position will be reintroduced to offset the nurse manager's increased workload. However, no one was able to describe the impact of this on the intended budget savings associated with expanding the nurse manager's responsibilities.

Patient Care Quality

Very little was learned during this site visit with regard to the impact of change on patient care. Around 1989 a patient satisfaction survey pointed to problems for the hospital, including in the nursing area. The CNO stated that when the need for budget reductions increased in the early 1990s, the decision was made to stop doing the patient satisfaction survey, even though she tried to indicate that this was the time for having even a better understanding of how the budget reductions might be affecting patient satisfaction. After a three-year lull, it was decided to conduct another patient satisfaction survey. Neither the nursing services nor the hospital fared well. The results of this survey prompted steps to be taken to increase nurse staffing and to implement some of the programs identified earlier by the CNO.

The CNO repeatedly indicated that someone needs to be identified as the responsible person in the organization for quality, and the CEO suggested the same. In addition, nurse managers expressed concern that the changes in their role might impact negatively on patient outcomes. In response to a question concerning the implications for the staff of the nurse manager's absence, one nurse manager said: "I think that what would occur with our staff is, and I've seen this, . . . [that] they would not buy into our cycle or outcomes. They would become frustrated, and you would probably have a higher turnover rate with our staff. Poor quality in regards to the clinical part. I don't think our patients or customers would get the quality that they needed to get." Another nurse manager answered: "They [nurses] need to have trust that someone's going to hear their concerns and to help them get where they want to be, and I don't mean personally, but with patients."

Again, this discussion reflects anticipatory change more than actual change. It is, however, representative of the nurse manager's perception of the ultimate impact of their role on patient care. Working with and through clinical nursing staff to establish the environment for high-quality patient care is the traditional responsibility of the on-site nurse manager. As nurse managers assume responsibilities that distance them from the operations of the clinical unit, the concerns they raise about the eventual loss to patient care quality somehow need to be addressed in the restructuring process.

CONCLUDING REMARKS

The story of the CNO's changing role at Blue Hospital is one filled with ambiguity. Learning to manage staff within a nursing practice model that empowers the clinical nursing staff for decision making along with the managerial nursing staff has begun only recently. The nursing staff do not yet fully understand the impact of that kind of change on an organization and on patient care, yet they are about to embark on a new organizational structure and care delivery system that is certain to change, in part, some of the new design recently implemented in the nurse manager and associate director role responsibilities. Whether the professional development sought by the nursing department can be achieved within the compressed time frame now available remains to be seen, particularly given the conditions of additional and much larger organizational change. And, if it cannot be achieved, what are the implications for patient care in the future?

Thanks to the CNO's work, nursing has started to be recognized at Blue Hospital. The CNO is perceived by the clinical nursing staff and managers to have taken a number of risks to make changes that have helped them in their work. However, ambivalence about the level of nursing's influence was voiced by senior members of the administrative team at both the hospital and corporate levels of the organization. The CNO herself indicated that she had a difficult beginning in the organization because she lacked a good working relationship with the previous CEO. The result was that she felt undermined by others and experienced difficulty with her peers.

It was clear that changes were occurring in the CNO role that were subtle and may not be understood as yet by staff. In preparation for the changes soon to occur, the CNO was diminishing her leadership role for nursing in the organization. Clearly, the CNO designer role is dominant at this time. Less evident were the integrator and communicator roles. Some evidence of the liaison role spoken of by Mintzberg (1973) is found in the CNO's increasing responsibility for the organization in more outside activities, especially in speaking and traveling. It seems that there may be interest at the system level in increasing nursing leadership, although this too is confusing and has yet to unfold in the restructuring process. Moreover, expansion of this CNO's role at that level continues to be undetermined.

In many ways, Blue Hospital seems to be striving to reach a model for nursing and patient care that many other hospitals already have found in the past decade. At the same time, it has put in place an ambitious plan for overall restructuring of the patient care system that will impact directly and significantly on the traditionally central role of a nursing department within the hospital.

7

Contextual and Thematic Findings

"As nurses assume the role of corporate officer, they will assume other departments and all of the fiscal power that goes with it. . . . As the job expands . . . what is relinquished? What are the implications for organizational structure?"

—M. A. Poulin

This study does not pretend to answer the question Poulin posited in 1984 as she concluded the report of her examination of the structure and function of the CNO role in hospitals. Instead, her question is used here to note the evolutionary nature of change. As expected, change itself is an overriding finding of this qualitative research study aimed at examining the CNO's changing role in the midst of a larger sea of change. Using the analytical framework set forth in chapter 3, this chapter explores the impact of change on clinical operations, especially as related to nursing services, and identifies the themes that emerged from the cross-study examination of the three case studies discussed in chapters 4, 5, and 6.

CONTEXTUAL VARIABLES THAT INFLUENCE THE CNO ROLE

The CNO role is influenced by numerous contextual variables, including those of job and the individual. These contextual findings, and the thematic findings discussed in the second part of this chapter, form the basis for the response generated from this study to the four study questions discussed in chapter 3.

Environmental and Situational Variables

Although many people perceive the Clinton administration as having failed in its effort to pass health reform legislation, the debate that effort sparked has helped to initiate incredible change in hospitals and health systems throughout the country. As the data obtained from the three study sites suggest, the major overall catalyst for change has been health care financing policy.

There were striking resemblances in the sites studied as well as obvious differences. Each of the study hospitals is part of a larger system trying to position itself within an increasingly competitive health care market. Although only one site was dealing with the complex issue of becoming one hospital as a result of a merger, all three were heavily involved with larger system issues related to acquisitions, affiliation, or competition with multiple other health facilities.

The managed care ratio of each hospital's revenue, excluding non-HMO Medicare, was similar—26 to 30 percent—with the expectation that it will increase in the near future. Similar also was the recognition by all three hospitals that they were facing ongoing financial pressure to reduce costs. The need to accelerate cost-reduction efforts was a key consideration in their attempts to address other important issues such as organizational structure and role expectations.

Organizational Structure   At the time of the study visits, all three hospitals were involved in restructuring their core delivery system for patient care. Again, both similarities and differences were found in their efforts. For example, all three had a similar overall approach to organizational restructuring and work redesign: a form of product line restructuring for the reorganization of clinical services, and a patient-focused care approach to their work redesign efforts. However, despite the similarity, their results are different, representing three distinct organizational patterns for the management of nursing and patient care services:

- Hospital-based, staff-level management
- Partial administrative management of product lines
- Complete product line management

The difference in these patterns is best described by the presence or absence of central leadership for nursing or for patient care services in general.[1] Organizationally, the difference is expressed by the pattern of change found in the CNO role. The patterns discussed in table 1-3, in chapter 1, were supported by this study in general, although none appeared exactly as suggested in that discussion.

Particularly significant was that a hospital-based, staff-level CNO role was not anticipated to be one of the patterns. A staff, rather than a line, role for the CNO position was considered to be a potential at the system level of the organization, but not at the hospital level. This pattern was found in Red Hospital's postmerger reorganization. Additionally, the CEO of Blue Hospital strongly suggested that in the future the CNO role would become a staff administrative role, ostensibly similar in design to that in place at Red Hospital.

This raised the question of the permanency of the current structures; perhaps they are transitional only. If so, for how long? How stable does an organization need to become following major change before introducing another major change that directly affects the relationships of those individuals who provide its core services? These were questions raised but not answered by the data found in this study.

Another unexpected finding relating to the assumed prestudy CNO role patterns was the administrative management of product lines by CNOs, substituting, in part, for management of the department of nursing. The model of product line services, some of which are managed by the CNO, was found at White Hospital and Blue Hospital, and a strong product line management structure exists at Red Hospital, which divides responsibility among vice presidents who happen to be nurses but are not organizationally sanctioned as senior leadership roles for nursing.

Initially, it was thought that expansion of the CNO's administrative line responsibilities was taking place through the development of an inclusive patient care department encompassing nursing and other discipline-specific departments (social service, rehabilitative services, pharmacy, and so on). A totally combined patient care service department such as this was not found in any of the three hospitals, although each of the CNOs had individual members of other disciplines reporting to them. Both the literature and anecdotal information suggest, however, that the model of an inclusive patient care department is structurally in place at other hospitals.

The conventional departmental approach to the hospital's organizational structure for nursing was found at Blue Hospital only, and as previously discussed, that structure has since been changed to product line management. Preparation for this change was ongoing at the time of the site visit. White Hospital has retained a nursing service component in its patient care service and product line approach. But Red Hospital has eliminated any essence of a central departmental approach to the clinical operations of nursing except for professionally related functions, most of which are provided to others in the organization on request. This incremental demise of nursing services as a central department of clinical operations was one of the most dramatic changes found in this study, the impact of which is described in the discussion of themes later in this chapter.

Role Expectations of the CNO   The emerging organizational models found highlight the hospital's changing nature that was discussed in the literature review for this study. To what extent is the hospital moving from a professionally oriented organization to a business-oriented one? Helping to integrate the hospital's two traditional organizational structures—administrative and clinical—has been a central component of the CNO role, providing balance and direction for others and designing patient care systems to support such integration. Product line management emphasizes attention to the business and economics of care delivery in a different way than the conventional organizational models do. It is assumed that the focus of the CNO managing these product lines will change as well. The demands of managing product lines are bound to consume the CNO's attention, raising the question: How much time will the CNO have left to develop creative strategies for clinical discipline leadership?

The need to pay attention to the business side of care delivery is not in question. What is in question is the potential choice of one value over the other. This is what concerns many health care professionals. At what point does a change to a financial- and business-focused orientation in the delivery of services overturn the balanced distribution of a professionally oriented influence on the hospital's strategic direction and decision making?

In the early twentieth century, the internal balance of power of hospitals changed significantly when the financing of hospitals moved from total reliance on the benevolence of community trustees to greater reliance on payments from patients, thereby indirectly expanding the sphere of influence of physicians in hospitals (Starr 1982). Today, it appears that another shift in the balance of power is taking place, again the result of changes in hospital and health care financing. The full consequence of this redistribution of influence is unknown, and the balance of power is yet to unfold. Ultimately, the indicator of that balance will be found in the outcomes of patient care.

Job- and Person-Related Variables

Although individual CNO attributes were not a focus of this study, their impact cannot be separated from the study findings. Leadership is part of structure. Consequently, throughout the study analysis, the style and substance of each CNO's leadership indicated the important impact that variables associated with the individual can have on organizational outcomes.

The only person-related variables centered on during the interviews were those of a demographic nature. Table 7-1 displays a profile of the CNOs who participated in this study. All were female, married, and of the same approximate age and educational background, which suggested that their entrance into nursing was at a similar generation of professional development.

Although all three participating CNOs had graduate degrees, only one had an advanced degree in nursing (as well as a second master's degree in health administration). During the interviews, each CNO stated her belief that the CNO needed to have an advanced degree outside nursing in order to compete on a level ground with other administrators. However, the CEOs interviewed immediately identified a clinical background as an essential element of CNO educational preparation and were likelier to suggest that some combination of a clinical and business degree was needed. These two perspectives on the educational preparation needed for effective CNO functioning probably reflect the CNO's role expectations to balance issues related to both the administrative and clinical tracks of the hospital organization.

CNO Tenure   The interviews revealed a difference in the tenure of the CNOs participating in the study. The most tenured CNO was located at Red Hospital, where she now holds a staff, rather than a line, position. The least tenured CNO, located at White Hospital, has retained, within her line of

TABLE 7-1. CNO Profiles

	Red Hospital	White Hospital	Blue Hospital
Organizational Title			
—Current	Vice president of clinical support services and CNO	Vice president of patient care	Vice president of patient care services and CNO
—Former	Vice president of nursing	Vice president	Vice president of nursing
Educational Preparation			
—Diploma, nursing	Yes	Yes	Yes
—BS, nursing	Yes	Yes	Yes
—Master's, nursing	No	No	Yes
—Master's, other (health administration or MBA)	Yes	Yes	Yes
CNO tenure (this hospital)	24 years	$1\frac{1}{2}$ years	9 years
Age	56	53	50
Gender	Female	Female	Female
Marital status	Married	Married	Married

authority, more central leadership for both nursing and patient care. As discussed in the case study of Red Hospital, tenure probably played a small part in the decisions made relating to the redesign of the CNO role. However, there was no evidence to suggest that tenure is a decision-making variable generalizable to other organizations.

However, tenure is a variable that can be related to role relationships and work behaviors (Mintzberg 1973). A new CNO has not yet developed relationships and much of her work includes building a network that will assist in providing needed information. The CNO's liaison and disseminator roles are particularly important during this initial period in the position. This accounts, in part, for the work relationships developed by the CNO at White Hospital. As a new person in the position, she needs to establish her own network in order to be effective in the required roles of communicator and integrator. Because all the CNOs in this study basically are new to their role (or, as at Blue Hospital, moving to a new role), rebuilding a network of relationships should be an important dimension of the work they now do.

Title as Status Symbol   Symbols of status are found in all organizations, but perhaps the most universal of these is that of position title. Titles provide some insight into the job function, but even more than that, they suggest hierarchy, status, and, ultimately, role partners and organizational relationships (Newcomb, Turner, and Converse 1965; Mumford and Skipper 1967).

The designation of CNO was held by each of the senior nursing leaders interviewed in this study. The organizational title held was that of a vice president, suggesting their placement at the senior level of the organization. This was the title more prominently identified in the two organizations where the CNOs continued in a line position. In the past, the CNO designation generally has not been a visible part of the organizational title. Previously, there was no necessity to use this designation overtly because the identity of nursing was incorporated within the official position title. Now, as titles and role responsibilities expand for the CNO position, nursing's visibility as a discipline no longer may appear to exist at the executive level of the organization unless the CNO designation is embodied in the title. The extent to which this designation is embraced as part of the position title may relate to the incumbent's personal choice as much as anything. Will the incumbent's work identity be predominately as administrator of the organization, leader for the discipline, or both? It was the assumed need for the discipline's visibility at the executive level of the organization that led the AHA board of trustees to include nurse administrators (CNOs) on the senior leadership team (AHA 1983).

As discussed throughout this book, the change in organizational identity has caused concern among nurse managers and other nursing leaders who fear the loss of their discipline's voice at the senior level of management. These concerns are similar to those voiced by nurses during the two national nursing shortages of the 1980s. During that time, clinical nursing staff felt their concerns about the delivery of patient care services were not understood at the highest level of the organization. They wanted to ensure that the interests of the direct care provider were understood and included in the organization's decision-making process.

Concerns about Patient Care   Finally, an important similarity found among the CNOs interviewed was the interest they all expressed for and about patient care. They were committed and passionate in their discussion about maintaining the quality of care. Throughout the study, hope was expressed by the CNOs, clinical specialists directors, and CEOs interviewed that the CNO would remain a patient advocate, an interest that also was articulated by all three CNOs.

THEMATIC FINDINGS

Across-site analysis of the case studies was performed to identify common themes. Five major themes emerged:

1. Boundary expansion
2. Transitions
3. Loss
4. Cohesiveness
5. Power shifts

Although treated independently for the purpose of discussion, it should be pointed out that these themes are interrelated and not easily separated or prioritized into isolated notions.

For some of these data, the thematic grouping was arbitrary. Perhaps it could be argued that material designated in one theme category could be designated just as easily in another. Overlap of theme data was experienced throughout the analysis, with some data seeming to represent more than a single theme.

As previously noted, change is an overriding theme incorporated into the body of discussion of the five major themes identified. One other theme emerged in a similar way—conflict and ambiguity. Because this theme was such an integral part of the other themes, it is included below as part of their discussion rather than being treated in isolation.

Boundary Expansion

Boundaries are part of an organization's dynamics, in part representing the beginning or end of authority and responsibility. Generally, boundaries are sanctioned by the position held and the scope of responsibilities assigned. Gilmore (1988) indicated that it is the role of leaders to take up positions on boundaries, mediating as necessary. In essence, Mintzberg's (1973) liaison leader role (or integrator, as categorized for this study) relates to boundary management, providing purpose, as Gilmore says, within the context of the whole.

Multidimensional Boundary Expansion   In this study, boundary expansion was found to be multidimensional, furnishing both breadth and depth to the CNO's role responsibilities. However, this finding was not limited to the CNO. A surprising finding was the extent of boundary expansion within the nurse manager role as well.

No single pattern can be described for boundary expansion. Differences were found within each hospital as well as across the three hospitals. The generalities that can be described about role and boundary expansion are those that relate to product line (service line) management and patient-focused care.

Interdisciplinary and Interdepartmental Teaming   There is a far greater emphasis on interdisciplinary and interdepartmental teaming, for both the planning and implementation of services. The time pressures placed on the system as a result of the hospital's financial constraints have led to this important change in work functioning. The management boundaries of many nurse managers, once limited to nursing personnel only, now often include management of all those whose services have been decentralized to the patient care unit level. These services range from those of other clinical disciplines, such as social service, pharmacy services, and rehabilitative services, to those of other departments, such as transportation, housekeeping, and materials management. Even without having management authority and responsibility for these areas, boundary spanning through interdisciplinary and interdepartmental work has become an essential part of the work requirements of all, especially the nurse manager.

Managing members of other disciplines or areas was found to be a part of the nurse manager role even if the CNO's responsibilities do not incorporate these same services. As experienced in this study, the pattern of nursing management no longer trickles down the organizational hierarchy in the exact form as it once did. The breadth of management can be narrow or wide at any level of the organization, and does not need to be an exact duplicate of the other.

Boundary Expansion for the CNO   The study findings did not provide a clear direction for generalizing boundary expansion for the CNO. One CNO (White Hospital) held virtual responsibilities, across the organization, wherever patient care existed, although her management responsibilities were not as broadly defined. At the same time, the depth of her responsibilities for programs and operations was being expanded as she assumed total administrative responsibility for selected product lines. As CNO of White Hospital, she has complete authority as well as responsibility to carry out the three roles of integrator, communicator, and designer for nursing and patient care services.

At Blue Hospital, the direction the CNO role was about to take was less clear at the time of the interviews. However, it now appears that boundary expansion relates to product line management and responsibility for other clinical departments such as pharmacy. Nursing as a department no longer exists, nor did it seem that a central component of nursing services would remain in the same fashion as at White Hospital. Central leadership for nursing is expected to occur through a professional council of representative members of the nursing staff led by the CNO.

The CNO at Red Hospital was in a clearly diminished role in terms of overall organizational responsibilities and influence. Her communicator role had been curtailed significantly, especially in terms of being a disseminator of information, a critical component for fulfilling the other important role of integrator. Absent was the organizational status needed to interact with others as a sanctioned leader for the purpose of both getting and giving information. Her access to clinical and managerial nursing staff is limited because her staff role does not provide the needed legitimate base of power to use the resources of the collective nursing staff. Personal influence only is the base from which she is able to operate.

Systemwide Involvement   The CNOs and nurse managers in all the study hospitals are involved in the larger systemwide issues, but, not surprisingly, each role participates in different ways. For each CNO, membership on a systemwide Council of Nurse Executives was expected, and all three are involved in other system-level committees or planning retreats. Nurse managers, on the other hand, are involved more directly in meetings with clinicians from different parts of the system, planning clinical services across the continuum for a specific product or service line. The meetings are interdisciplinary, and the nurse managers feel obligated to represent the discipline of nursing. As discussed in the section on loss, nurse managers have conflicting feelings about this new responsibility.

Transitions

Gilmore (1988) noted that leadership transitions in organizations provide a natural time for change because of the destabilization that occurs simultaneously. The theme of transitions was found across all three study sites. For the most part, the transitions related to the CNO's leadership role and the changes stemming from reorganizing the hospital's management structure.

Transitions surface much ambiguity in the organization, whether resulting from the installation of a new CNO, as at White Hospital, or anticipating implementation of a new structure and organizational design, as at Blue Hospital. Not knowing what to expect next caused one nurse manager to suggest they were all floundering.

At Red Hospital, transitional ambiguity resulted from the tremendous overall void in leadership present because of the interim nature of so many of the senior leadership positions, including the chief executive office. The CNO, normally the person nursing staff looked to for direction and clarity of purpose, now was a confusing role within the organization. The transition of this role from its traditional central leadership position for a very large segment of the hospital's employee population to one of no central leadership was unsettling for many.

Because leaders are expected to help absorb the uncertainties in an organization, the transition of leadership found at each of the study sites was especially significant. Transitions are important times in the life cycle of an organization and can provide opportunities for rebuilding and learning new skills, as well as for creating new leadership teams. The CNO's communicator role should become as important as ever during a transition, not only for exchanging needed factual information but also for using this time of destabilization to inculcate values and purpose. The investments made, or not made, during this unique transitional time will shape future patterns for the organization (Gilmore 1988).

Loss

Perhaps the most emotionally intense theme found was that of a sense of loss. This was repeated throughout the three organizations and at all levels. But none of the descriptions of loss were as intense as those given by nurse managers and other clinical nursing leaders.

Once again, identity symbols within the organization were spoken of in terms of loss by the nurse managers and clinical leaders. The lack of an identifiable nursing department and the change of titles that no longer provide external recognition of the nursing discipline were elements of the discussions held throughout the three settings. However, these conversations paled in comparison to those of nurse managers describing the changes they perceive to have occurred in the relationships they now have with their CNO and their own staffs

Trust and Distance   Two commonalities were found in the theme of loss. The first relates to distance and the second to trust. These are discussed together because of the difficulty in extracting one from the other. An important function the CNO has performed in hospitals is that of bringing to the administrative decision-making table a central voice for the concerns nurses and other clinicians have related to patient care delivery. In doing so, the CNO conveys, in some ways, the voice of the patient and the family. Fulfilling this role expectation is more than simply being a nurse. Opportunities to interact with those in the direct line of delivering service must be in place; being able to get and give information through organizationally sanctioned interaction with others allows the roles of integrator, communicator, and designer to be actualized.

In each of the settings visited, nurse managers and others interviewed expressed the feeling that this central role of the CNO was either already lost or at risk of being lost. The reasons for these perceptions differed across settings, but the intensity with which those closest to the delivery of care expressed their concern was the same. The nurses' need to trust that someone who understands their practice is advocating at the highest levels of the organization for what they do on behalf of patients and families was repeated in every interview with nurse managers and others involved in the direct line of caregiving. In two groups, a similar statement of concern was expressed from the single individuals representing other disciplines—respiratory and physical therapy. The central nature of nursing, serving within the organization as the nexus for all patient care services, was underscored again through these discussions.

Changes in the CNO role functions have led to changes in the relationships the CNOs have with the nurse managers as well. In all three hospitals, a strong concern was voiced about the growing distance between CNO and nurse manager. Whether the change was actual or symbolic did not matter; the distancing was felt. Central meetings with the CNO through which a cohesive approach to care delivery could be formed were viewed in all settings to have diminished as other changes occurred. In the view of nurse managers, this translated into a loss of common vision or direction that eventually would be realized in the quality of patient care provided. This disconnection between nurse manager and CNO was complicated by another organizational change occurring in the role of nursing director.

In each hospital, the change to a product line approach for the organization of clinical services has changed the middle manager nursing role of nursing director. In some cases, the span of control for nursing directors has increased, as many have assumed the position of either director of patient care services or product line manager. Although, technically, they are still responsible for the nurse manager, like the CNO, the time they spend individually and collectively with nurse managers is substantially less.

In some ways, the disconnection between nursing director and nurse manager is a more severe loss than the disconnection between nurse manager and CNO. Nursing directors have been the link between nurse managers and CNOs, helping to move forward the common vision and goals by nurturing and supporting the frontline clinical managers. Loss of this continuous nurturing was spoken of by all groups of nurse managers interviewed. They no longer had someone who could support their ideas about the work or who would help them reflect on problems and issues requiring attention.

Complicating this was the finding that the nurse manager's own span of control had increased substantially. Some have found their workload expanded as they accept responsibility for managing more than one patient care unit. Even those who had not yet had their responsibilities expanded beyond one unit believed that it was only a matter of time before this would occur. The discussion of their changing relationship with nursing directors, coupled with the fact that there now are fewer assistant nurse manager positions, made their anxiety about workload expansion understandable. The CNOs confirmed the changes in workload level and number of nurse manager FTEs. Table 7-2 displays, by hospital, the change in the number of nurse manager positions. It should be noted that some nurse manager deletions relate to the actual closing of units.

As discussed in the earlier section on boundary expansion, many of the nurse managers interviewed have assumed cross-system responsibilities, representing the nursing component of clinical service integration and development. This has brought another level of time commitment into their work schedules, which was a point of fervent discussion.

Role Conflict   Many of the nurse managers were conflicted about the extension of their responsibilities beyond the operational management of patient care units. As mentioned earlier, they now interface with many other disciplines across the system, in some cases more often than the CNO does. On the one hand, they have a different level of personal challenge they like and believe has been helpful in learning more about the work of others. They feel up to the work and, for the most part, enjoy the opportunity to engage in planning for services with others in this way. However, they also feel a great deal of conflict. They recognize that the

TABLE 7-2. Change in Nurse Manager FTEs, by Hospital

	Red Hospital	White Hospital	Blue Hospital
Nurse managers			
No. of FTEs, 1991–1992	75	29.8	31
No. of FTEs, 1995–1996	51	21	24

depletion they are experiencing by not having the same opportunities they once did for ongoing nurturing and mentoring from either the nursing director or the CNO is the same issue clinical nursing staff are experiencing. They are frustrated that the clinical nursing staff they once felt professionally close to now express concern for not having the consistent on-site leadership presence they need from the nurse manager. In profound ways, nurse managers were more concerned about the separation that has occurred in their relationship with the clinical nursing staff than about their expanded workloads.

This finding has great significance for CNOs and others involved in designing new paradigms for the organization and the future management of clinical services. The expertise of the on-site clinical manager is invaluable in the planning process of clinical services. The CNO is limited in this technical expertise and must rely on the specialists. At the same time, the on-site support and development provided to clinical staff from this same expert clinical nurse manager are fundamental in achieving the patient care outcomes desired. New designs calling for clinical and managerial partnerships are in order and need to be sought.

Finally, the theme of loss raises concerns beyond those described. If new organizational designs are developed without a strong central CNO voice for nursing, is it possible that the organization has increased its vulnerability for union activity? The concern of nurses that they are losing the voice of nursing at the senior level of organizational decision making can be offset, in part, by having strong on-site nurse manager–clinical nurse relationships. If the perceived distance between management and clinical staff found in this study occurs across a larger segment of the hospital field, there is a greater possibility than before that clinical staff will seek an alternative voice and an increase in collective bargaining activities with nurses could be the result. In all the hospitals visited, including the one whose nursing staff was already unionized, the potential for a union response to changes made was suggested by either the CNO or the CEO. Clearly, this would constitute an unintended consequence of restructuring.

Cohesiveness

Cohesiveness—defined by the *American Heritage Dictionary* as a logical, orderly relationship of parts—surfaced as a separate theme as the interview content related to loss was reexamined. Interrelated with the theme of boundary expansion, nurse manager concerns that new structures were leading to fragmented systems of patient care suggest that the loss they felt was more than personal. They no longer perceived themselves as a collegial, professional group developing a common direction for high-quality patient care.

Restructuring has dismantled the conventional central mechanisms for discussing and communicating issues of patient care. Problem solving leading to hospitalwide standards of care was considered compromised without this centrality. The product line approach, although considered useful in improving interdisciplinary work within the clinical service, was viewed as problematic because of the organizational isolation that seemed to result. Each product line had its own hierarchy, standards, and priorities. The patterns of communication between them were viewed as complex, leading to a level of concern about how overall standards of care would be implemented and monitored. The conventional departmental organization relied on the functioning of a central nursing department to help others understand the impact of change on others. Restructuring to a decentralized clinical management organization seems to have changed the vertical silos of departments to horizontal silos with cumbersome systems of communication.

Power Shifts

Closely related to all the other themes discussed is the concept of organizational power shifts. Underlying many discussions were hints of change in the management interests of physicians as they also respond to a changing work environment. Signs of this were seen in the organizational placement of more physicians in administrative roles, particularly ones associated with quality improvement. To a large extent, this was viewed favorably by those interviewed. However, some were concerned that the interests of individual physicians would take precedence over the interests of other clinicians, leading to a further decline in a common direction for patient care.

The ability of nurses to act effectively when they no longer form a cohesive group also emerged in the discussions. The lack of a unified approach across all patient care components of the organization was viewed as problematic. If patient care standards became dependent on the resources of the individual product line, inconsistency in patient care across the hospital could result. Nurses have relied on the CNO role to reduce the organizational barriers that lead to results such as these.

Power shifts also are occurring within the ranks of nursing. Concurrent with the dismantling of an organized, discipline-specific departmental approach, individual nurses have gained greater influence in both the clinical and administrative tracks of the hospital. In two of the hospitals, for example, nurses other than the CNO hold senior-level leadership positions. This is well received, but because of the nature of their administrative functions, their placement in the organization does not provide an adequate substitute for the professional dimensions of unity that emanate from a community of nurse colleagues striving to achieve a common vision.

SUMMARY OF RESPONSES TO THE STUDY QUESTIONS

To a large extent, the four study questions developed to guide this qualitative study of the impact of restructuring on the role of the CNO and nursing management in hospitals already have been answered in this chapter. This section summarizes the contextual variables and thematic findings discussed above.

1. Is the CNO Role Changing from the Traditional Focus of Setting-Based Practice to One of an IDS Practice?

A CNO position at the system level of the IDS was not found in any of the three study sites visited. However, nursing involvement was found at the system level in various forms. A nurse executive council exists in each of the systems, which suggests that a cross-system focus on nursing is desirable. The CNO of each of the flagship hospitals participates as a member of her respective council. The agenda for these councils varied and related to common issues of nursing and patient care services as generated by the CNO participants or issues delegated to them by other components of the system-level structure. With regard to the latter, the most common activities delegated to this group related to quality improvement projects.

Other, systemwide activities were found to occur in the CNO role, but only on a limited basis. The focus of CNO responsibility remains within the hospital, and there is some evidence that it has begun to encompass the continuum of services to patients and families.

Involvement at the system level of other members of the nursing management team, especially the clinical nurse manager, was found to be occurring. This involvement is mostly interdisciplinary and focused on clinical service integration across the system.

2. Has the CNO Role Evolved from a Discipline-Specific Focus (That Is, the Nursing Service) to One of Broader Accountability for Patient Care and the Continuum of Services?

At all the sites visited, the designated CNO was involved in organizational issues that encompassed a broader scope of responsibility than that of the discipline focus of nursing alone. Designing systems for patient care that encompass continuum of care needs was found to be incorporated within the CNO role functions. However, no single direction was found in the pattern of CNO accountability for a comprehensive patient care service. All CNOs were found to have other disciplines within their scope of responsibility, but none had responsibility for a consolidated patient care service department.

Managing members of other disciplines or other departments was more likely to be found in the clinical nurse manager role responsibilities. Expansion of the responsibilities of this organizational position was more than had been anticipated and served as a pivotal component of the discussion of thematic findings.

3. Is the CNO Role Incorporated into the Organization's Executive Level?

Once again, the direction found in this study is unclear. All three CNOs held an executive-level title of vice president and attended senior-level administration meetings. At one hospital, the level of CNO participation at the executive table was considered to have increased substantially in recent times, whereas, in another, CNO involvement was far less substantive than in the past. The breadth of CNO involvement at the third hospital was unclear from the information gathered during the site visit. Executive involvement by the CNO probably is a combination of the variables of situational context, job elements, and elements that are person related.

4. Have Changes in the CNO Role or Hospital Organization Had an Impact on the Management of Nursing Services?

This question is answered throughout the discussion of findings within each of the case studies, as well as in the cross-study analysis presented in this chapter. Substantial change was found in the design of the nursing services as well as the design of the managerial roles in nursing. An identifiable central nursing department is no longer evident in the restructured hospital. One symbol of this change is the absence of the nursing discipline as an organizational element on the hospital's organizational chart. More significant is the concern that this represents a loss of a central place for developing consistency in patient care standards and care practices.

There were diminishing numbers of nurse managers, directors, and assistant nurse managers found in each of the hospitals. Changes in the CNO role had cascading effects on other managerial roles, especially in terms of diminishing contact as organizational structures change and communication patterns are altered. The loss of a sense of direction and vision for patient care, usually provided by the CNO, was expressed by those interviewed.

One interesting result of the dismantling of the nursing department was learning the extent to which others depend on it as their infrastructure for communication and for patient care system planning. At the heart of this nexus is the CNO.

Notes

1. The term *patient care services* is used to describe the collective services of most, if not all, clinical disciplines. Sometimes this includes management of all nonclinical services within the same administrative structure, but it also may represent a conceptual framework for organization or a virtual organizational model.

8

Implications for the Future

O ver the years, the position of CNO, now often called either vice president for nursing or vice president for patient care services, became increasingly influential within hospital organizations, making a difference not just in the practice of nursing but also in the quality of patient care. However, as the hospital industry began to address issues such as cost reduction, managed care, mergers and affiliations, and IDS development, it became clear that the CNO position would experience change. And it was the desire to examine the change in this position that prompted the study described in this book.

Although the study was expected to reveal changes in the CNO role, the substantial structural change in the department of nursing services found at the three sites was unanticipated. Additionally, during the study interviews, it became evident that change was occurring not only in the CNO role but also in other nursing leadership roles within the organization, especially in the nurse manager role.

The study findings support what is well known in the current health field environment—that change is abundant and that the process of change seems to be accelerating. Because this is a time of such transition, new patterns for conventional roles such as that of the CNO are emerging. The patterns themselves may be transitional, serving as bridges for a future organizational design still unknown. This chapter looks at some of the implications for future hospital policy that may be drawn from the findings of this study.

IMPLICATIONS FOR HOSPITAL POLICY

The findings of this study have implications for those involved in policy within health care organizations as well as for those in the field of nursing, selected regulators, and health policy researchers. The following discussion serves to highlight some of the areas for further policy analysis and research.

CNO Role

Although it is clear that the CNO role is changing, neither the direction nor the degree of change is evident. The study suggests that one potential change will be movement of the CNO position to a staff role within the hospital. For this to be at all effective, the CNO must be truly incorporated into the executive level of decision making and have open access to the nursing leadership positions across the organization. The CNO's role is to ensure that a common direction for patient care is developed and integrated with the goals of the organization. Without access to both the executive and nursing leadership levels, the potential for CNO leadership in a staff role is seriously compromised.

The study findings also show that other executive positions in the hospital are being filled by nurses, suggesting that as organizations change, nurses may be carrying out broader administrative responsibilities at senior levels. The study site CEOs often mentioned that the background that nurses bring to the administrative arena is needed during this time of expedient and turbulent change. Although these new executive roles do not necessarily provide the clinical leadership for nursing addressed in this study, their increasing prevalence may suggest that when the current cycle of change stabilizes, nurses will permeate all levels of the organization in many roles and not just those associated with management and leadership within the clinical discipline of nursing.

Although it is difficult to prescribe how any one organization should structure itself or how roles should be determined for the organization, this study does provide some information that can be used in making these decisions. Interview data from all three study hospitals suggest that a central locus of clinical leadership be maintained as restructuring occurs. However, the data also show that the changes in the clinical leadership component of the CNO role have not kept pace with the growth and strength in the administrative realm of that role. This distancing of the CNO's leadership role away from the professional domain of clinical nursing may ultimately have deleterious effects on nursing practice and, subsequently, patient care. Health care organizations should consider ways to structurally provide for professional interaction and clinical leadership by the CNO or a senior-level designee with clinical nursing staff.

Moreover, the lack of a consistent or standard meaning attached to the CNO designation is striking. Unlike CFO or CEO, the title of CNO does not carry the same understanding across settings or within the field itself, nor does it universally suggest executive-level functioning in the organization. The CNO *designation* can be found at all levels of the organization. Other roles are sometimes so designated merely to meet regulatory obligations. This diminishes the CNO identity within the field of health care, making the contributions of the role and the discipline far less visible and less influential, again to the potential detriment of patient care.

Perhaps the expectations of the nurse executive role as currently defined by the JCAHO should be revisited as part of an effort to determine how it is being implemented in the evolving health environment. In addition, the CNO designation should become standard, representing a particular function and level within the health organization. AONE should accept responsibility for leading these efforts in collaboration with the AIIA. A plan for reestablishing the CNO's executive-level placement and senior clinical leadership role for the discipline within the evolving health system should be developed.

Restructuring Process

Having a catalyst for change was an important part of the restructuring process in each of the hospitals visited. It was interesting to note the influence the national project funded by the Robert Wood Johnson Foundation and the Pew Charitable Trust had on motivating these hospitals toward a quality improvement project that ultimately led, in two of the hospitals, to a restructuring process. Although funding was helpful in developing the overall focus of quality improvement, it seemed to provide a crucial opportunity for people to take time to reflect on practice and exchange views on how patient care systems should evolve. Time for reflecting, examining practices, and determining direction has seldom been built into the operational management of dynamic services such as those provided by hospitals. The positive outcomes achieved by the hospitals that received a grant requiring a cross-system view of patient care suggests that this is a useful process for planning.

Workforce issues become a major consideration in the change process that is needed to transform hospitals into twenty-first-century organizations. Nurses, as well as other clinical workforce groups, generally have not worked as independently of others within their respective disciplines as these new structures are suggesting. Rather, their work has been as cohorts or as a community of caregivers. The cohesiveness and infrastructure long associated with a central leadership and management structure for nursing services have provided stability, particularly as a communication vehicle, for the work of nurses as well as other clinical and hospital groups. As this structure is dismantled, organizational chaos and workforce instability are major risks. One of the cataclysmic worries about breaking up the nursing department is the potential loss of an infrastructure that traditionally has provided a safety net for all of patient care. Those designing new organizational paradigms must consider these aspects of the structure, which for the most part have been taken for granted in the organization.

A lot of the new work of the emerging hospital system is interdisciplinary. For restructuring to be effective, one of the real needs in the change process is to help people focus on how to work together in an interdisciplinary and collaborative way. This calls for an examination of decision-making processes to ensure parity among professionals. Horizontal communication among peers and colleagues is needed for organizational effectiveness, regardless of department or product line structure.

And finally, the fragmentation of nursing in the newly designed patient care systems may stem from a fundamental flaw in the way nursing as a department has often been viewed within hospitals. The scope of CNO responsibility in each of the study hospitals was described by number of areas managed (mostly inpatient units) and by number of FTEs or size of budget. Perhaps conceptualizing the CNO responsibilities as leadership, both organizational and professional, for a clinical discipline, no matter the size or place of practice, would provide a different kind of framework and one that might prove to be more difficult to disregard regardless of the organizational design of clinical services.

View of Nursing as a Discipline

The way RNs are viewed within the health field has a lot to do with the way they are used within the hospital organization and elsewhere. If nurses are considered one of many different workforce inputs that simply support the medical profession or physicians in their practice, only one organizational model for nursing practice will evolve. However, if nurses are considered members of a clinical discipline who bring unique contributions to patient care outcomes, a different organizational model will emerge.

Nurses often find they need to reposition themselves and continuously defend their practice in order to achieve recognition as members of a distinct discipline. As organizational structures for patient care are dismantled and the potential risks or benefits of these changes to patients are yet to be learned, policy makers should not chance leaving nursing out of the policy-making process. Nursing needs to be recognized as a unique clinical discipline, and nurses must be invited routinely to participate with others in the determination of health care and organizational policy. As a first step, they should always be considered appropriate partners for collaborative work in the formulation of high-quality patient care standards that relate to the financing policies of health care. As the largest group of health care workers in the labor force, nurses represent a major economic health care investment that should be used wisely.

CNO Role Theory

How a role is implemented can depend as much on the interests and strengths of the individual in the role as on the job variables sanctioned organizationally. This suggests that there is a delicacy of roles that can put other components of the organization out of balance when the choices of the individual are permitted to supersede the needs of the organization. Some of the study findings suggest that changes in the CNO role may have been influenced substantially by the choices, styles, interests, and attributes of the incumbent CNOs. This raises interesting theoretical considerations in the continued study of the CNO role.

In a study of the executive influence of hospital CEOs, Chilingerian (1987) discussed the personal choice aspects of an executive's focus of attention. Tenure, information gathering and sharing, personal access and organizational influence, and network development were among the many areas of choice influencing the CEO's attention.

A similar question must be raised for this study. That is, how much of the CNO role change in the three study site hospitals relates to the individual in the job and what she chooses to attend to, and how much is out of her control or direct influence? The theory of personal choice should be further explored as changes in health care organizations continue to take place.

IMPLICATIONS OF THE FIVE THEMES IDENTIFIED

The five themes that emerged from the story of the change process within the three distinguished hospitals studied suggest a number of questions for the future. These are explored in the following sections.

Boundary Expansion

The study findings suggest that organizational boundaries are shifting away from the traditional department of nursing to an organizational structure in which nursing services are unidentifiable and integrated within the structure of product lines. Concurrent with this is evidence of a new homogeneity of clinical management at the nurse manager and senior nursing leadership levels. An expansion of management responsibilities appears to be taking place in all nursing management roles, raising important questions about the design of hospital management positions in the future. Will there be new boundaries managed by nurses only, or will these boundaries be open for generic clinical management by any discipline? And, most important, how will the chosen design affect patient care?

Examination of these questions might be enlightened by examining the experience of other professional groups. For example, as engineers became more highly integrated into their work organization, did they forfeit their professional identity and occupational culture? Is the blurring of nursing's identify different because of the historical and symbiotic nature of the practice of nursing and the hospital organization? In hospitals, is this change a prototype for what will happen with other professional groups, or is it limited to nursing?

Transitions

The effect of role transitions is evident in each of the organizations visited, as is ambiguity about these transitions. Reorientation of people from the old to the new must be understood by those making change as an important part of transition management, a concept to be differentiated from change management (Bridges 1988).

This study reveals that many different kinds of transitions are occurring besides those of role change for nursing management. However, these changes and those associated with organizational structure have the greatest meaning for those involved and the psychological transitions associated seem to be the most evident. It remains to be seen whether the current transitions are a part of real, evolutionary changes in hospital organizational structures or whether they are cyclical changes that, over time, will revert to some of the previous structures. In either case, their effect should be tracked through organizational research or evaluation measures, especially as they relate to the cost and quality of patient care.

Loss

Evidence of loss surfaces at all three sites in many different ways. Clearly nurses' loss of identity as a professional group is an uppermost concern, but the strongest concerns are related to those losses in the system that are perceived to have a potentially serious impact on patient care.

Because of the strong role the nursing service structure has played within hospitals as the nexus for patient care systems, an examination of the consequences of dismantling the nursing department should be undertaken. A lesson to be studied, perhaps, comes from the Chinese Cultural Revolution of the 1960s, which resulted in the obliteration of all the professions and their identity in Chinese culture. Now, as the Chinese wish to reorganize and move forward in a competitive world, they lack the professional resources required.

The questions that loss raises include

- What does the loss of central nursing leadership mean for other parts of the organization?
- What effect does it have on the autonomy of a professional group?
- What are the ultimate implications for patient care?

These questions should be examined concurrently with any proposed organizational changes.

Cohesiveness

The study participants reported that cohesiveness within the clinical staff and a common direction and vision for patient care were necessary elements in achieving the desired outcomes for patients and families. The vehicle for common direction is personal contact with senior-level leadership, which, in the hospital setting, has traditionally been the CNO. Also, patient care itself is a personal service relying on the nurturing of clinicians for effectiveness. These features also carry over to organizational relationships. The model of personal contact, nurturing, informing, and reflecting is one that nurses value in their own relationship with hospital leadership. It is the CNO who has carried out this role the best.

If nurse managers are to be distanced from their clinical product— patient care—careful studies must be done to evaluate the outcomes of such a significant change. Perhaps, in part, one way to right the system is to openly acknowledge that the work of the nurse manager has changed. During this time of transition, the new work of this managerial role should be focused, perhaps, on managing the organizational change process rather than on managing clinical care, as in the past. However, in doing so, the need to design a system that provides a focused resource for clinical care management also must occur. Designing new leadership roles for nurses who work in partnership may be one approach to achieving these equally compelling needs. Careful study of new models needs to occur.

One of the outcomes of the loss of a cohesive structure is a concomitant loss of opportunity for clinical practice development and advancement of the profession through scholarship. Where will or should this development, which has been so historically tied to hospital nursing practice, take place in the future? And if it is no longer considered an appropriate hospital function, are there consequences for patient care?

Power Shifts

Product line, a business and industrial model used for the marketing and differentiation of services or products, has been increasingly adopted for use in organizing hospital clinical services. This approach to the organization of clinical services began to be popularized in hospitals following implementation of the Medicare PPS and DRGs in the early 1980s. The intent is to become more efficient in the management and delivery of clinical services (Maarse, Rooujakkers, and Duzijn 1993).

The change to a product line management and organizational structure redistributes organizational power. Product lines are aligned primarily with the clinical services of medicine. The increased involvement of physicians associated with medical specialties in organizational management is part of this shift of power. In addition, a product line organizational structure decentralizes the hospital management structure in a way that often leads to the demise of discipline-specific departments. This is especially so for the nursing department.

Does the change to product lines upset the balance of organizational power in a way that is detrimental to patient care outcomes? Why is product line becoming such a popular organizing structure? Are there alternative models, or is product line the only organizational structure for the future? What elements of product line make this structure a preferred model?

FINAL OBSERVATION

It was not the intent of this study to examine the various restructuring efforts undertaken by hospitals, but rather to gain insight into the implications of those efforts on the clinical operations of the organization as it is viewed through the perspective of the chief nursing role. The study clearly points out the way restructuring, especially the change to product line, impacts on nurse managers and others in clinical leadership roles. This discussion of CNO and nursing management role change, however, could apply to other clinical disciplines practicing within the hospital. Thus, the study of the current change phenomena within hospitals may have implications for others as well. Social workers, pharmacists, and physical therapists are some of the other clinical disciplines beginning to experience changes similar to those discussed in this study. The experience of nursing provides, then, a useful example of the serious and multiple changes under way in hospitals and demonstrates the concerns for patient care that are raised by many clinical groups.

Within the lessons learned from this study are insights related to change itself: how and why organizations undertake change and the impact that organizational and external environmental factors have in determining the process of change. Among the many notable variables for change was the relationship of the CEO and CNO. Successful teaming of these two critical leadership positions was perceived by others in the organization to be an important component of success in developing good patient care delivery systems. This suggests that the position of CNO needs to be placed at the right level of the organization in order to ensure that the CNO has access to other appropriate role partners as well. The integration of clinical and administrative values and goals depends in large measure on the opportunities afforded by these relationships and cannot be minimized.

In light of the findings of Aiken, Smith, and Lake (1994), this suggests that patient care outcomes relate to the level of nursing autonomy—nurses' control over practice and physician relationships. Nurse managers' concerns of feeling distanced from the clinical staff should be considered very seriously when an expansion of the responsibilities of this role is contemplated. Part of the nurse manager's work is to help remove the barriers that prevent autonomous and collaborative nursing practice. Distancing the clinical nursing staff from the nurse manager could interrupt this process and lead to less desirable patient outcomes. Clinical and managerial partnerships might be useful in preventing this perceived distancing. That is, clinical nurse specialists and administrative managers working as partners with the nurse manager may be a way of strengthening the leadership team that supports the clinical staff, nursing as well as others.

Consideration should also be made of the means by which a central infrastructure for patient care services might be retained as decentralization to local units of service occurs. At a minimum, it appears that there remains a need for effective and well-coordinated patient care standards, quality improvement systems, and performance standards. The nurse executive role is the most likely senior leadership position to assume this accountability.

Lastly, this study was prepared to offer an information base to senior management and policy makers about the organization and management of the hospital as it positions itself within a restructured health care environment. As health care systems build new networks and develop new organizational roles in the future, the question of role, function, and boundaries of the chief nursing officer remains. The complexity of hospital restructuring suggests that clarity needs to occur in the conception of the chief nursing officer role and nurse executive positions.

The development of a standard definition of CNO, such as that derived from the work of Poulin and of Hunt (see chapter 1) might be useful in guiding organizational decisions around this senior-level leadership position. Perhaps also, the complexity of the health care systems calls for broader involvement of nurse executives at both the hospital and system level and requires multiple nurse executive positions in some organizations. One of these may also assume the designation and function of CNO. It may be that a CNO nurse executive position is needed at the system level, suggesting that the systemwide coordination of professional and clinical standards for nursing and patient care might take on a more significant role in the future as interdisciplinary and decentralized management models emerge within hospital settings. This design for nursing and patient care service integration at the system level could be a corollary to the systemwide physician integration efforts that are also taking place and might serve as a quasi-model for the interdisciplinary partnerships needed in the future.

These thoughts represent only some that might be considered as hospital restructuring continues to take place in the United States and even worldwide. Continuing to examine the implications of change, while also making a change, is a challenge in itself—but nonetheless a needed process. The changes suggested as a result of this study raise multiple questions for the clinical disciplines involved, including the ultimate and socially responsible question: In the end, what will these changes actually mean for patient care and the health status of our society?

Appendix A

The Role and Function of Nurses in Executive Practice

PREAMBLE

The purpose of this document is to clarify and communicate the evolving role of nurses in executive practice. Nursing focuses on the human health experience and is uniquely positioned to shape community care networks for healthy people.

The essence and values of nursing form the basis for all nursing roles and are the foundation for the advanced practice of nursing administration. The elements that guide nurse executive practice include

- Networks of wellness, acute care, ambulatory, and long-term care providers
- Collaboration among health professionals in interdependent functions
- Partnerships with consumers
- Collective accountability
- Advocate for those who cannot advocate for themselves
- Leadership in cost-effective patient care

TRANSITIONS

Nurses in executive practice are transitioning from traditional setting-based practice to integrated community-based practice. The role of nurses in executive practice has evolved from a focus on nursing services to a broader accountability for patient care services across the continuum. This expansion of role responsibilities places nurses in executive practice and other nurses in key leadership positions. The role transition reflects the following shifts:

- From provider-driven to consumer-driven systems
- From responsibility for episode of care to responsibility for health care throughout the life span
- From reactive to community or health needs to proactive for community or health service needs
- From process to balanced structure process and outcomes
- From a focus on disease treatment to a focus on prenatal care, wellness, prevention, rehabilitation, long-term and self-care, and alternative therapies
- From an individual consumer focus to a population and society focus
- From fee-for-service to capitated and managed care reimbursement methods

DIMENSIONS

1. Clinical processes
   —Standards development
   —Clinical integration
   —Consumer self-care and involvement
   —Continuity
   —Innovation
   —Community participation
   —Education, research, ethics
2. Leadership
   —Shared vision
   —Relationships
   —Organization ethics
   —Developing others
   —Change agents
   —Strategic thinking
   —Development through research
3. Continuous improvement
   —Decision making
   —Organizing
   —Resource (assessment, procurement, allocation)
   —Quality/cost accountability
   —Systematic outcome improvement

Key Processes of Nurse Executive Practice

- Facilitating the design of patient care delivery
- Advancing the discipline of nursing
- Building relationships and connections
- Facilitating transitions
- Positioning, representing
- Researching, developing, supporting
- Negotiating
- Fostering stewardship
- System integration

Enabling patients and communities, and their resources, needs, and problems, drive the evolution of the nurse executive role. Major themes in all the dimensions of this role are collaboration, diversity, cocreating, communicating and coordinating, outcomes management, and enabling the spirit of the community.

SUMMARY

Within the continuum of nursing executive practice, there exists varying titles, shifting positions, and an evolving dynamic configuration of function(s). Expression of the dimensions vary in emphasis by scope of accountability and focus of practice. The accountability for the respective role must be commensurate with the position in the organization and the resources to accomplish this work. Shifts in emphasis can be best illustrated on a continuum of practice from the point or unit of patient care delivery to the system. Influencing, direction setting, designing the processes for care delivery, and system development broaden in scope along this continuum. However, due to the uniqueness of the evolving organizations and communities developing community care networks, this process is not occurring linearly, but in a dynamic, interactive, and integrative fashion.

This document was developed by the AONE Commission on Practice and was reviewed and refined by the membership in spring 1995.

Appendix B

Interview Guide

O verall focus: What is happening? Why is it happening? What are the implications?

Intent of Questions	*Interview Content Sought*

Introductory, demographics, and general discussion of CNO role and any changes	• Title of CNO. Any recent or expected changes?
	• Tenure of CNO.
	• Changes in the CNO role in recent times (that is, the last three years).
	• What differences in:
	  —Meetings
	  —Budget and financing participation
	  —Strategic planning
	  —Nursing activities
	  —Patient services
	  —Management
	• What prompted the change in this role?
	• Is CNO role changing more than other roles?
	• Role of CNO in network or system activities.

(Continued on next page)

Intent of Questions	*Interview Content Sought*
CNO relationships and accountability; clinical practice development for nursing, for others, and for improving the quality of patient services and care	• What changes have occurred in the management and organization of nursing services? • How are they perceived to have affected: —Patient care —Morale —Relationships with nurses —Other departments • How visible is the CNO to nursing staff and others? Communication opportunities—how designed? • Changes in quality of care? • What opportunities for nurses to interact with the CNO? Has this changed? With other departments? • Have changes in the CNO role impacted the role of other nursing management positions?
How is the CNO incorporated into the executive level of organization?	• Reporting relationships of the CNO. • Who is considered the peer group of the CNO? • What is the CNO's relationship with: —Hospital administration/board —Physician leadership —Nursing staff —Other departments • CNO involvement in strategic planning? in the implementation? • How is the CNO's role described as part of the hospital? the system? • What committees, councils, or other forums does the CNO participate in on a regular basis? —Medical staff leadership —Board of trustees —Executive leadership

Appendix C

Letter to the CEO*

May 1996

Dear [CEO],

Along with my role as the Chief Nurse Executive at Beth Israel Hospital in Boston, I am also a PhD candidate at the Heller School of Social Welfare and Health Policy at Brandeis University, Waltham, Massachusetts. In this latter role, I am at the dissertation stage of my studies.

The purpose of this letter is to ask for your willingness to allow [your hospital] to be one of the three flagship hospitals of three integrated health care systems participating in this study. The focus of my study is the changing role of the chief nursing officer in the current health care environment. I have enclosed an abstract of my study for your review.

Because case study analysis is the methodology being used, your willingness to participate involves engaging in an interview with me for approximately two hours. The purpose of this interview is to glean your view, as the CEO, of the chief nursing officer role. I also request participation of the chief nursing officer of [your hospital]. This interview is designed to elicit information about the structure and role relationships of the chief nursing officer, not performance of the CNO.

It may be necessary for me to follow up by way of a phone call should there be any portion of the interview that will need further clarification. Consent to participate in this study, therefore, may involve a follow-up phone call no longer than one hour. I will also seek general demographic information about the hospital, an organizational chart, and position description of the chief nursing officer.

It is my hope that [your hospital], as a leading institution in the changing health care environment, will participate in this study. (Your name was provided to me as the hospital CEO along with the name of the CNO.) If you confirm that this is the chief nursing officer that should be contacted for participation in this study, I will do so by phone and a follow-up letter.

It is my hope to be able to visit [your hospital] for this purpose sometime in June. Ideally, I would interview you as well as the chief nursing officer on the same day. Each interview would last approximately two hours. It does not matter which interview occurs first and, if necessary, I would stay another day in order to complete both interviews in this single trip.

I will call your office soon to determine your willingness to participate in this study and, if so, a date and time suitable for you and the chief nursing officer. Your signature on the enclosed copy of this letter serves as informed consent. You can return it to me by mail, or I will pick it up during my visit to your hospital. I look forward to hearing from you and appreciate your consideration of this request.

Sincerely yours,

Joyce C. Clifford, RN, MSN, FAAN

---

*Parts of this letter have been edited from the original to preserve the anonymity of the participants.

Appendix D

Letter to the CNO*

May 1996

Dear [CNO],

Thank you for agreeing to have me visit [your hospital] on June __, 1996. As the enclosed letter to [the CEO] indicates, I am interested in interviewing you and [the CEO], as well as other appropriate persons for the purpose of examining organizational change as hospitals respond to the increasing climate of managed care and integrated delivery systems. The focus of the organizational change is the chief nursing officer role, and the changing management and administration of nursing services in the acute care hospital. I have enclosed an abstract of my proposal for your use as well.

In preparation for my visit, there are some materials that would be helpful for me to have—ideally in advance of my arrival. But if that is not possible, I will pick them up when I am with you. Because my interest is in tracking the change that is happening, I am interested in receiving both a current and prior (3–5 years ago) copy of each of the following documents:

- A table of organization for the hospital and for the nursing services.
- The position description of the chief nursing officer and of other significant positions if you think they are applicable to my study.
- Chief nursing officer responsibility for budget and FTEs (that is, current FTE responsibility as percent of hospital total and the same information for 3 to 5 years ago). If possible, can these data be provided as number of RNs, other nursing personnel, and then others described by appropriate major categories such as social workers, physical therapist, and so on (assuming they now are included in the changed responsibilities of the CNO). It is not my intent to have you rework your systems to provide me this information, so whatever form you have such data in will be

acceptable for me. I can ask for any clarification when I talk with you.

I am also interested in having a general profile of the CEO and the CNO. If you and [the CEO] are willing to share your CVs with me, that would be helpful. In general, what I want to know is: (1) how long you each have been with this organization, (2) how long you have been in your current position, and (3) your educational preparation.

I hope this is not an imposition. I know what busy and hectic times all of us are now engaged in and although I am most interested in learning as much as possible about your organization and the changes you have made and are making, I do not want to add a burden of work to anyone's day.

As we discussed by phone, I would also like to meet with a group of nurse managers and any other group or individual you think would be useful for this study. I will ask only for permission to use a tape recorder in order to capture the full richness of the discussion I expect to find. If there is anything specific you would like me to share with you or others about the Beth Israel Hospital, I will be happy to do so; let me know. Clearly, when the analysis of [your hospital] is completed, I will share the results with you.

Your signature on the enclosed copy of this letter serves as your consent to participate in this study, as well as the consent of those you will ask to join me in any discussions. If there is a different procedure you prefer to have me complete, please let me know. I can pick up your signed copy during my visit in June.

I am truly looking forward to this opportunity and again thank you in advance for your willingness to participate in this study.

Sincerely,

Joyce C. Clifford, RN, MSN, FAAN

---

*Parts of this letter have been edited to preserve the anonymity of the participants.

References

Abdellah, F. G. 1970. *Overview of Nursing Research, 1955-1968.* Rockville, MD: National Center for Health Services Research and Development.

Aiken, L. 1990a. "Charting the Future of Hospital Nursing." *Image* 22 (2): 72–77.

Aiken, L. H. 1990b. "Letter to the Editor." *Health Management Quarterly* 12 (1): 3.

Aiken, L., H. Smith, and E. Lake. 1994. "Lower Medicare Mortality among a Set of Hospitals Known for Good Nursing Care." *Medical Care* 22, no. 8 (August): 771–87.

Altman, S. H. 1971. *Present and Future Supply of Registered Nurses.* Washington, D.C.: U.S. Government Printing Office, DHEW Publication Number (NIH) 72–134.

American Hospital Association. 1983. *Future Directions: Report of the Board of Trustees.* Chicago: AHA.

American Hospital Association. 1994. *Restructuring Health Care Delivery: Legal and Common Terms.* Chicago: AHA.

American Nurses Association. 1974. *Facts about Nursing 72–73.* Kansas City, MO: ANA.

American Society of Nursing Service Administrators. 1977. *Survey of Nursing Service Administrators in Hospitals.* Chicago: ASNSA.

American Society of Nursing Service Administrators. 1982. *Survey of Nursing Service Administrators in Hospitals.* Chicago: ASNSA.

AONE. 1995. "The Role and Function of Nurses in Executive Practice." Chicago, Ill.: AONE.

ASHHRA/OMNI. 1995. *Semi–Annual Labor Activity Report, 7th Report, Jan. 1, 1995–June 30, 1995.* Chicago, Ill.: The Omni Group, Inc.

Ashkenas, R., et al. 1995. *The Boundaryless Organizations: Breaking the Chains of Organizational Structure.* San Francisco: Jossey–Bass, pp. 1–30.

Baloga, M. 1993. "Role Expectations of Chief Nurse Executives." *Dissertation Abstracts International* 31 (4): 1, 728.

Benveniste, G. 1987. "Beyond Bureaucracy: Why Profession–Oriented Organizations Are More Effective." In *Professionalizing the Organization.* San Francisco: Jossey–Bass, pp. 254–70.

Bergman, R. L. 1993. "Quantum Leaps." *Hospitals & Health Networks* 67 (19): 28–35.

Berwick, D. 1994. "Eleven Worthy Aims for Clinical Leadership of Health System Reform." *JAMA* 272 (10): 797–802.

Beyers, M. 1994. "Is the Nurse Executive Role Expanding or Contracting? *Journal of Nursing Administration* 24 (11): 8–9.

Beyers, M. 1988. "The Nurse Executive Role in Not-for-Profit Multi-Institutional Systems." *Series on Nursing Administration* 1, 71–99.

Biester, D. 1994. "Creating a Professional Nursing Work Environment: A Story of Organizational Transformation." *Dissertation Abstracts International* 55 (5): 1, 799.

BJC Health System. 1996. *BJCTODAY* 2 (1).

Blau, P. M., and W. R. Scott. 1962. *Formal Organizations.* San Francisco, CA: Chandler Publishing.

Boyce, R. A. 1992. "The Organizational Design of Hospitals: A Critical Review." *A Report of the Australian College of Health Service Executives Overseas Study Award.* College Monograph no. 1. NSW, Australia: Australian College of Health Service Executives.

Brannon, R. L. 1994. *Intensifying Care: The Hospital Industry, Professionalization, and the Reorganization of the Nursing Labor Process.* Amityville, NY: Baywood Publishing.

Bridges, W. 1988. *Surviving Corporate Transitions.* Mill Valley, CA: William Bridges & Associates.

Buerhaus, P. I. 1996. "Understanding the Economic Environment of Health Care." In *The Managed Care Challenge for Nurse Executives.* AONE Leadership Series. Chicago: AHA.

Burner, O. Y. 1983. "The Organizational Structure of Air Force Hospitals and Its Effect on Management of Nursing Services." *Dissertation Abstracts International* 43 (7): 2,431A.

Carroll, N. V., and W. G. Erwin. 1987. "Patient Shifting as a Response to Medicare Prospective Payment." *Medical Care* 25 (12): 1, 161–67.

Chilingerian, J. 1987. "The Strategy of Executive Influence: An Analysis of the Attention Structure of the Hospital Chief Executive Officer." PhD diss., Boston: MIT.

Christman, L. P., and M. A. Counte. 1981. *Hospital Organization and Health Care Delivery.* Boulder, CO: Westview Press.

Cilliers, G. J. 1989. "The Expected Leadership Role of Nursing Administrators." *Nursing Administration Quarterly* 13 (3): 47–54.

Clifford, J. C. 1981. "Managerial Control vs. Professional Autonomy." *Journal of Nursing Administration* 9, 19–21.

Clifford, J. C. 1985. "The Nurse Executive in the Institution's Leadership Team." *World Hospitals* 21 (4): 28–30.

Cohen, J. H. 1989. "Nurse Executives' Psychological Well–Being: The Relationships among Stress, Social Support, Coping, and Optimism." *Dissertation Abstracts International* 49 (DAI–B 50/05, November 1989): 1,850.

Colburn, D. 1994. "Nurses' Jobs Are Changing or Disappearing." *Washington Post*, November 22, 1994, pp. 7–8.

Colloton, J. W. 1984. "The Future Role of the Nurse Executive: To Make a Difference." Presentation to the Boston University Graduates of the Commonwealth Fund Executive Nurse Leadership Program, Boston, November 1984.

Cowley, G., S. Miller, and M. Hager. 1995. "Intensive Care on a Budget." *Newsweek*, February 13, 1995, p. 86.

Crossley, J. D. 1993. "Chief Nursing Officer Governing Body Proximity, Direct Reporting Relationship, and Professionalism as Predictors of Chief Nursing Officer Role Conflict and Role Ambiguity." *Dissertation Abstracts International* 54 (4): 1, 887B.

Davidson, S. M., M. McCollom, and J. Heineke. 1996. *The Physician–Manager Alliance: Building the Healthy Health Care Organization*. San Francisco: Jossey–Bass.

Davis, C. K., P. D. Powell, and M. S. Gross. 1987. "The Changing Health Care Environment." *Topics in Health Care Financing* 14 (1):1–8.

Davis, F., ed. 1966. *The Nursing Professional: Five Sociological Essays*. New York: John Wiley & Sons.

Davis, N. K. 1989. "Relationship of Organizational Culture and Leader Effectiveness of the Nurse Executive." *Dissertation Abstracts International* 49 (DAI–B 50/04, October 1989): 1,323.

Department of Health and Human Services. 1988. *Secretary's Commission on Nursing, Final Report*. Vol. 1. Washington, D.C.: U.S. Government Printing Office.

Dock, L., and I. Stewart. 1925. *A Short History of Nursing*. New York: G. P. Putnam and Sons.

Duke, D. S. 1996. "Hospitals in a Changing Health Care System." *Health Affairs* 15 (2): 49–61.

Dunham, N. C., D. A. Kindig, and R. Schulz. 1994. "The Value of the Physician Executive Role to Organizational Effectiveness and Performance." *Health Care Management Review* 19 (4): 56–63.

Edwardson, S. R., and P. B. Giovannetti. 1987. "A Review of Cost Accounting Methods for Nursing Services." *Nursing Economics* 5 (3): 107–17.

Eisenhardt, K. M. 1989. "Building Theories from Case Study Research." *Academy of Management Review* 14 (4): 532–50.

Etzioni, A. 1964. *Modern Organizations*. Foundation of Modern Sociology Series. Englewood Cliffs, NJ: Prentice–Hall.

Etzioni, A., ed. 1969. *The Semi–Professions and Their Organization: Teachers, Nurses, Social Workers.* New York: The Free Press.

Ferguson, V. 1989. "The Nurse Executive: Comfort and Presence." *Journal of Professional Nursing* 5 (6): 298.

Finer, H. 1952. *Administration and the Nursing Services.* New York: The Macmillan Co.

Freidson, E., ed. 1971. *The Professions and Their Prospects.* Beverly Hills, CA: Sage.

Georgopoulos, B. S., ed. 1972. *Organization Research on Health Institutions.* Ann Arbor: The University of Michigan, Institute for Social Research.

Gilmore, T. N. 1988. *Making a Leadership Change: How Organizations and Leaders Can Handle Leadership Transitions Successfully.* San Francisco, CA: Jossey–Bass Publishers.

Gilmore, T. N., L. Hirschhorn, and M. O'Connor. 1994. "The Boundaryless Organization." *Healthcare Forum Journal* (July/August): 68–72.

Ginsburg, P. B. 1996. "The RWJF Community Snapshots Study: Introduction and Overview." *Health Affairs* 15 (2): 7–20.

Glesne, C., and A. Peshkin. 1992. *Becoming Qualitative Researchers.* New York: Longman.

Greene, J., and S. Lutz. 1996. "A Tale of Two Ownership Sectors." *Modern Healthcare* 26 (no. 21, May): 61–74.

Greiner, A. 1995. *Cost and Quality Matters: Workplace Innovation in the Health Care Industry.* Washington, D.C.: Economic Policy Institute.

Hansen, M. C. 1993. "Perceptions of Chief Nurse Executive Competencies." *Dissertation Abstracts International* 54 (3): 1, 332B.

"Health Care Reform: Nursing's Vision of Change." 1993. *Hospitals* (April): 20–26. (Mundinger).

Henry, B., S. Woods, and J. Nagelkerk. 1992. "Nightingale's Perspective of Nursing Administration." *Nursing and Health Care* 11 (4): 201–6.

Hoechst Marion Roussel, Inc. 1995. Managed Care Digest Series. *HMO–PPO Digest*, p.16.

Hunt, J. M. 1994. "Excellence in Nursing." An unpublished report of a Nursing Research Initiative for Scotland.

Hurst, D. K. 1995. *Crisis and Renewal: Meeting the Challenge of Organizational Change.* Boston: Harvard Business School Press.

Hyndman, K. J. 1993. "Leadership in Nursing Administration: The Perspectives of Senior Nurse Administrators." *Dissertation Abstracts International* 32, no. 2 (April): 596.

Interstudy Competitive Edge. 1996. *Part III: Regional Market Analysis, Reporting Data as of July 1, 1995.* St. Paul, MN: Interstudy Publications.

Jeska, S. B. 1994. "Luminous Leadership: A Qualitative Study of Nursing Administration Practice." PhD diss., University of St. Thomas.

Johnson, J. B. 1981. "The Relationship between Leader Behavior and Job Satisfaction as Perceived by Registered Nurses in Acute Care Hospitals." *Dissertation Abstracts International* 42 (6): 2, 404A.

Jones, K. R. 1989. "Evolution of the Prospective Payment System: Implications for Nursing." *Nursing Economics* 7 (6): 299–305.

Kanter, R. M. 1989. "The New Managerial Work." *Harvard Business Review* 67 (6): 85–92.

Katz, A., and J. Thompson. 1996. "The Role of Public Policy in Health Care Market Change." *Health Affairs* 13 (2): 77–91.

Kelly, J. 1977. "The Role of the Top Level Nurse Administrator." In *University of Minnesota Proceedings, Nursing, Administration: Issues for the 80's—Solutions for the 70's.* Minneapolis, Minn.: W. K. Kellogg Foundation, p. 157.

Knaus, W. A., E. A. Draper, D. F. Wayne, and J. E. Zimmerman. 1986. "An Evaluation of Outcomes from Intensive Care in Major Medical Centers." *Annals of Internal Medicine* 104, 410–18.

Kong, D. 1994. "Nurses Say Patient Feeling the Pain of Staffing Cutbacks." *Boston Globe*, October 31, 1994, pp. 37–38.

Koska, M. T. 1989. "Quality—Thy Name Is Nursing Care, CEOs Say." *Hospitals* 32, 32.

Kramer, M., and L. Hafner. 1989. "Shared Values: Impact on Staff Nurse Job Satisfaction and Perceived Productivity." *Nursing Research* 38, 172.

Kramer, M., and C. Schmalenberg. 1988a. "Magnet Hospitals: Part I: Institutions of Excellence." *Journal of Nursing Administration* 18 (1): 13–24.

Kramer, M., and Schmalenberg, C. 1988b. "Magnet Hospitals: Part II: Institutions of Excellence." *Journal of Nursing Administration* 18 (2): 11–19.

Kulbok, P. 1982. "Role Diversity of Nursing Administrators: An Obstacle to Effective Leadership?" *Nursing and Health Care* 3, 199–203.

Lathrop, P. 1992. "The Patient-Focused Hospital." *Healthcare Forum Journal* (July/August): 17–21.

Lawrence, P. P., and J. W. Lorsch. 1969. *Organization and Environment*. Homewood, Ill.: Richard D. Irwin.

Lowe, R. 1994. "Swapping over Roles." *Nursing Management* 1 (3): 18–19.

Lumley, D. D. 1988. "Decision Making in Hospital Nurse Executives: An Exploratory–Descriptive Study." *Dissertation Abstracts International*.

Maarse, H., D. Rooijakkers, and R. Duzijn. 1993. "Institutional Responses to Medicare's Prospective Payment System." *Health Policy* 25 (3): 255–70.

Massachusetts Hospital Association/Massachusetts Organization of Nurse Executives. 1995. *Report of Nursing Survey 1994*.

Mauskch, H. 1966. "The Organizational Context of Nursing Practice." In F. Davis, ed. *The Nursing Profession: Five Sociological Essays*. New York: John Wiley & Sons.

McClure, M. L. 1989. "The Nurse Executive Role: A Leadership Opportunity." *Nursing Administration Quarterly* 13 (3): 1–8.

McClure, M. L., et al. 1983. *Magnet Hospitals: Attraction and Retention of Professional Nurses*. Kansas City, MO: American Nurses Association.

McLemore, S. D., and R. J. Hill. 1965. *Management–Training Effectiveness: A Study of Nurse Managers.* Austin, TX: University of Texas, Bureau of Business Research.

Merton, R. K. 1957. *The Structural Context of Reference Group Behavior: Role Sets, Status Sets and Status Sequence, in Social Theory and Social Structures.* Rev. ed. Glencoe, Ill.: The Free Press, pp. 368–86.

Merton, R. K. 1968. *Social Theory and Social Structure.* New York: The Free Press.

MHA/MONE. 1996. *Report of Nursing Survey 1995.*

Mintzberg, H. 1973. *The Nature of Managerial Work.* New York: Harper and Row.

Mintzberg, H. 1989. "The Professional Organization." In *Mintzberg on Management.* New York: The Free Press, pp. 173–95.

Moses, E. 1992. *The Registered Nurse Population: Findings from the National Sample Survey of Registered Nurses* (U.S. Government Printing Office 0–16–042626–2). Rockville, MD: Health Resources Services Administration, Bureau of Health Professions.

Moses, E. 1984. *The Registered Nurse Population: Findings from the National Sample Survey of Registered Nurses* (NTIS Accession no. HRP–0906938). Rockville, MD: Health Resources Services Administration, Bureau of Health Professions.

Mullane, M. K. 1959. *Education for Nursing Service Administration: An Experience in Program Development by Fourteen Universities.* Battle Creek, MI: W. K. Kellogg Foundation.

Mumford, E., and J. K. Skipper Jr. 1967. *Sociology in Hospital Care.* New York: Harper and Row.

Nadler, D., and M. L. Tushman. 1989. "Organizational Frame Bending: Principles for Managing Reorientation." *Academy of Management EXECUTIVE* 3 (3): 194–204.

National Commission on Nursing. 1983. *Summary Report and Recommendations.* Chicago: The Hospital Research and Educational Trust.

Newcomb, T., R. Turner, and P. E. Converse. 1965. *Social Psychology: The Study of Human Interaction.* New York: Holt, Rinehart and Winston.

News Analysis, 1996. Melbourne, Australia.

Palmer, I. S. 1983. *Florence Nightingale and the First Organized Delivery of Nursing Services.* Washington, D.C: American Association of Colleges of Nursing.

Poulin, M. A. 1972. "A Study of the Structure and Functions of the Position of the Nursing Service Administrator." PhD diss., Columbia University, New York City.

Poulin, M. A. 1984. "The Nurse Executive Role: A Structural and Functional Analysis." *Journal of Nursing Administration* 14 (2): 9–14.

Prescott, P. A. 1993. "Nursing: An Important Component of Hospital Survival under a Reformed Health Care System." *Nursing Economics* II (4): 192–99.

Princeton, J. C. 1993. "Education for Executive Nurse Administrators: A Data-Based Curricular Model for Doctoral (PhD) Programs." *Journal of Nursing Education* 32, no. 2 (February): 59–63.

Reverby, S. M. 1987. *Ordered to Care: The Dilemma of American Nursing, 1850–1945.* New York: Cambridge University Press.

Riessman, C. 1993. *Narrative Analysis. Qualitative Research Methods, 30.* Newbury Park, CA: Sage.

Robinson, J. C. 1994. "The Changing Boundary of the American Hospital." *Milbank Quarterly* 72 (2): 259–75.

Rosenberg, C. E. 1987. *The Care of Strangers: The Rise of America's Hospital System.* New York: Basic Books.

Ryan, S. A. 1990. "A New Decade of Leadership: From Vision to Reality." *Nursing Clinics of North America* 25 (3): 597–604.

Schensul, J., and S. Schensul. 1990. "Ethnographic Evaluation of AIDS Prevention Programs: Better Data for Better Programs." In: L. C. Leviton, A. M. Hegedus, and A. Koelrin, eds. *New Directions for Program Evaluation.* San Francisco: Jossey–Bass.

Seidman, I. E. 1991. *Interviewing as Qualitative Research.* New York: Teachers College Press.

Seymer, L. R. 1957. *A General History of Nursing*. 4th ed. London: Faber and Faber Ltd.

Seymer, L. R. 1954. *Selected Writings of Florence Nightingale*. New York: Macmillan.

Sherer, J. L. 1993. "Physician CEOs: Ranks Continue to Grow." *Hospitals & Health Networks* 67 (9): 42.

Shortell, S. M. et al. 1993. "Creating Organized Delivery Systems: The Barriers and Facilitators." *Hospitals and Health Services Adminstration* 38: 447–66.

Shortell, S., et al. 1994. "The Performance of Intensive Care Units: Does Good Management Make a Difference?" *Medical Care* 32 (5): 508–25.

Shortell, S. M., R. R. Gillies, and K. J. Devers. 1995. "Reinventing the American Hospital." *Millbank Quarterly* 73 (2): 131–60.

Simms, L., S. Price, and S. Pfoutz. 1985. "Nurse Executives: Functions and Priorities." *Nursing Economics* 3, 238–44.

Singer, Charles J., & Co. 1996. *The Marketing Overview*. Wakefield, MA: Charles J. Singer & Co.

Society for Ambulatory Care Professionals. 1994. "Glossary of Managed Care Terms. In *Issue Briefing*. Chicago: SACP.

Sovie, M. D. 1995. "Tailoring Hospitals for Managed Care and Integrated Health Systems." *Nursing Economics* 13 (2): 73–83.

Starr, P. 1982. *The Social Transformation of American Medicine*. New York: Basic Books.

State Health Reform. 1992. "Five Trends That Will Transform Hospitals." *Hospitals* 66 (no. 19, October 5): 28–38.

Strauss, A. 1966. "The Structure and Ideology of American Nursing: An Interpretation." In F. Davis, ed. *The Nursing Profession: Five Sociological Essays*. New York: John Wiley & Sons, pp. 60–108.

Strauss, A., and J. Corbin. 1990. *Basics of Qualitative Research: Grounded Theory Procedures and Techniques*. Newbury Park, CA: Sage.

Tax Equity and Fiscal Responsibility Act of 1982 (Pub. 97–248). In *Prospective Payment Assessment Commission* (March 1, 1990). Report and Recommendations to the Secretary, U.S. Department of Health and Human Services. Washington, D.C.: Prospective Payment Assessment Committee, p. 15.

Tjosvold, D., and R. C. MacPherson. 1996. "Joint Hospital Management by Physicians and Nursing Administrators." *Health Care Management Review* 21 (3): 43–54.

Tribe, J., and D. G. Campbell. 1993. "A Proposal to Pilot Organizational Reforms." Unpublished report of the Royal Melbourne Hospital, Australia, June 1993.

Tubbesing, B. A. 1980. "Perceptions of the Director of Nursing Role in Hospitals." *Dissertation Abstracts International* 41 (5): 1, 719B.

Tucker, E. 1992. "Ethical Dilemmas of Nurse Executives: A Descriptive Study." *Dissertation Abstracts International* 52 (7): 3, 524.

Twedt, S. 1996. "Is a Cheaper Hospital Staff More Costly?" *Pittsburg Post–Gazette*, February 11, 1996, pp. 3–7.

VHA. 1996. *The Impact of Organizational Redesign on Nurse Executive Leadership, Part II: A Survey of Nurse Executives.* Second Survey Fall 1995. Texas: Voluntary Hospital Association, Inc.

Wangsness, S. I. 1991. "A Study of Decision-Making Activities of Nurse Executives in Acute Care Pennsylvania Hospitals." *Dissertation Abstracts International* 52 (4): 1, 939B.

Watson, J. 1995. "Advanced Nursing Practice . . . And What Might Be." *Nursing and Health Care* 16 (2): 78–83.

Watson, J. 1990. "The Moral Failure of the Patriarchy." *Nursing Outlook* 36 (2): 62–66.

Wilson, C. K. 1992. *Building New Nursing Organizations: Visions and Realities.* Frederick, MD: Aspen.

Witt Associates. 1990. *Today's Nurse Executive: Data Analysis, 1990 Survey.* Chicago: American Organization of Nurse Executives.

Witt Associates. 1986. *Today's Nurse Executive: Report of a Survey.* Chicago: American Organization of Nurse Executives.

Witt Associates. 1988. *Today's Nurse Executive: Report of a Survey.* Chicago: American Organization of Nurse Executives.

Witt/Kieffer. 1995. *Senior Nurse Executives in Transition: New Roles and New Challenges.* Chicago: American Organization of Nurse Executives.

Woodham-Smith, C. 1951. *Florence Nightingale, 1820–1920.* London: Constable and Co.

Workman L. L. 1995. *CGEAN Newsletter,* January 1995.

Wunderlich, G. S., F. A. Sloan, and C. K. Davis. 1996. *Nursing Staff in Hospitals and Nursing Homes: Is It Adequate? A Report of the Committee on the Adequacy of Nurse Staffing in Hospitals and Nursing Homes, Division of Health Care Services, Institute of Medicine.* Washington, D.C.: National Academy Press.

Yin, R. K. 1994. *Case Study Research: Design and Methods.* 2d ed. Thousand Oaks, CA: Sage.

Index

(Continued on next page)

151